THE
EASY MASSAGE
WORKBOOK

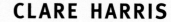
CLARE HARRIS

THE
EASY MASSAGE
WORKBOOK

A COMPLETE MASSAGE CLASS IN A BOOK

DUNCAN BAIRD PUBLIS

LONDON

The Easy Massage Workbook
Clare Harris

First published in the United Kingdom and Ireland in 2006 by
Duncan Baird Publishers Ltd
Sixth Floor
Castle House
75–76 Wells Street
London W1T 3QH

This edition first published in 2010

Conceived, created and designed by Duncan Baird Publishers

Managing Editor: Grace Cheetham
Editor: Rebecca Miles
Managing Designer: Manisha Patel
Designer: Rachel Cross
Commissioned Photography: Matthew Ward
Commissioned Artwork: Debbie Maizels

British Library Cataloguing-in-Publication Data:
A CIP record for this book is available from the British Library

ISBN: 978-1-84483-882-0

10 9 8 7 6 5 4 3 2 1

Typeset in TradeGothic
Colour reproduction by Colourscan, Singapore
Printed by Imago, Singapore

PUBLISHER'S NOTE
The information in this book is not intended as a substitute for professional
medical advice and treatment. If you are pregnant or are suffering from any
medical conditions or health problems, it is recommended that you consult a
medical professional before following any of the advice or practice suggested in
this book. Duncan Baird Publishers, or any other persons who have been involved
in working on this publication, cannot accept responsibility for any injuries or
damage incurred as a result of following the information, exercises or therapeutic
techniques contained in this book.

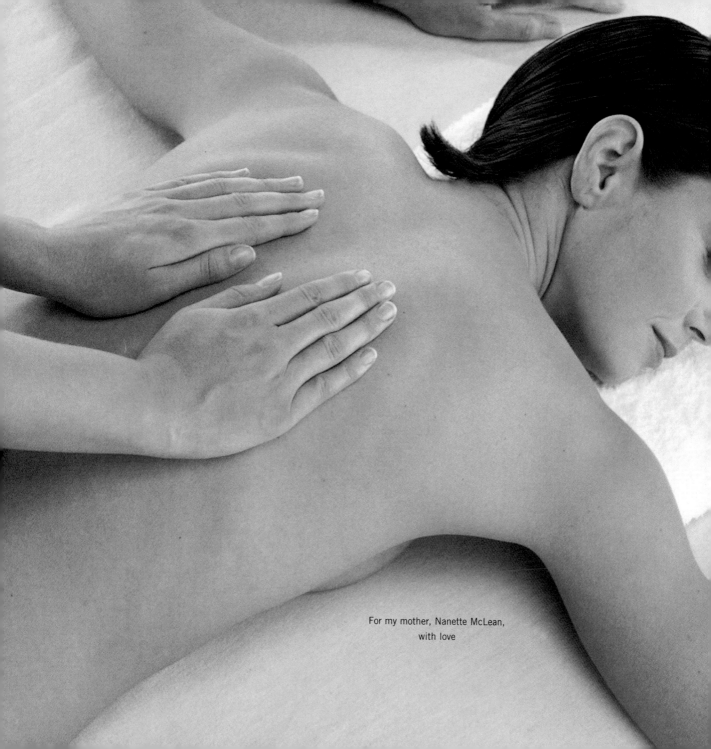

For my mother, Nanette McLean,
with love

Contents

SYMBOLS USED IN THIS BOOK

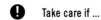 Massage stroke is good for ...

Take care if ...

Avoid if ...

Author's introduction

Twenty-five years ago when my children were small, I signed up for an evening class to learn massage. To my great disappointment, the class was cancelled before it began, because someone decided it was "an improper use of public funds". Later on, I found somewhere else to learn, and have been learning ever since. Over the last quarter-century, our knowledge and understanding of the physical and emotional benefits of massage has been transformed. It has been my privilege to play a tiny part in that transformation.

I came to understand that all of us hold our own patterns of chronic tension in our bodies, and that these physical-tension patterns usually mirror emotional tension and strain. Often we don't realize how much tension we hold until there is the time, space and privacy to have a trusted person's hands begin to stroke and knead that tension away. It is quite lovely to see what a transformation this can bring. The benefits of massage are increasingly well-researched; the immediate, positive effects on well-being are nothing short of astonishing — all from simple, skilful touch.

It may surprise you, as it did me, to discover what a deep personal satisfaction there is in giving a massage. You will find that your touch is healing to the person who is receiving it; at first you won't really believe this but it's true. I encourage you to use this book to explore different easy-massage techniques and routines, and to build your confidence. In time, your hands will "know" what is needed.

How to use this book

This book contains all the information you need to learn how to give a variety of good, simple massages. Before you begin to try these out, I suggest you first read chapter 1, which provides essential underpinning for all your learning. It includes an outline of what massage can do, when you are advised not to massage, how to prepare yourself and your room, and how to develop your awareness of both yourself and your massage partner.

Chapter 2 shows you nine massage techniques, which can be adapted for different areas of the body.

Chapter 3 gives you different massage routines, all of which can be used individually (such as the routines for the back or for the feet), or which you can link together to create a full-body massage.

Chapter 4 suggests some variations of what you have learned so far, so that you can adapt your massage work to suit different needs: for example, when massaging babies, pregnant women or the elderly.

Chapter 5 shows you how to use your new skills for yourself as well as others, offering simple self-massage routines to help with everyday minor ailments.

Finally, chapter 6 introduces you to some of the glorious range of oils you can use for massage: you will learn how to choose and store oils, and how to begin making beautiful aromatic blends.

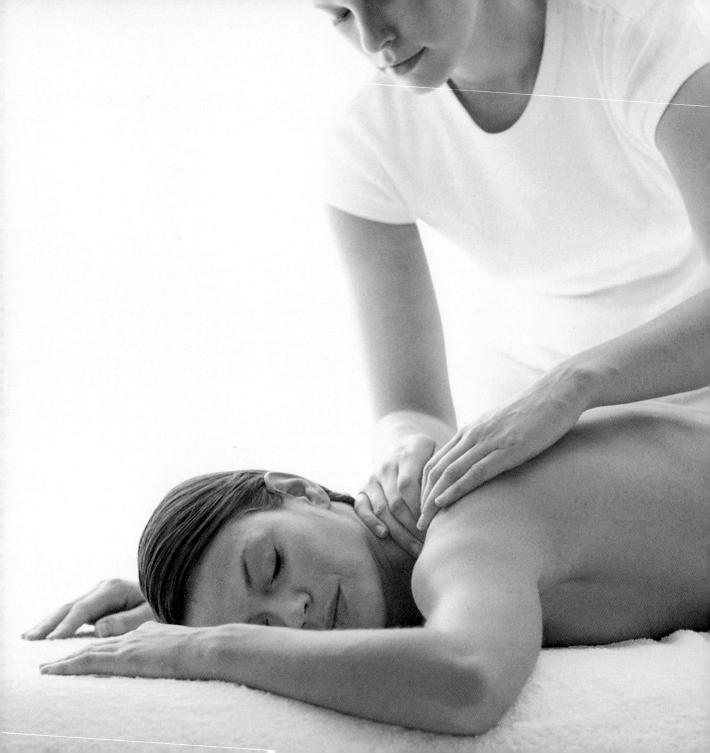

CHAPTER 1:
Easy Principles

Massage is an ancient form of healing that has been used over many centuries to relax, to comfort and to promote general well-being. It is a wonderful treatment to give as well as to receive. You don't need to be an expert to give an effective massage: even a simple ten-minute shoulder massage can have a transforming effect on the person receiving it.

This chapter gives you all the information you need to understand what massage can do and how it has been used through the ages. I will show you how to prepare for giving a massage, how to work with the body systems, and when you should take particular care. You will practise how to focus not only on your partner but also on yourself, so that, by the end of any massage you perform, your partner is relaxed and energized, and so are you.

What massage can do

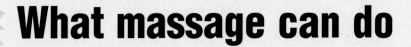

We are born needing touch. As babies the way we are touched and held is crucial for our little bodies to relax and blossom. As we grow into children, and become teenagers and then adults, the touch of another person can offer crucial support just when we need it, whether in the form of comfort during worry or sadness, a hug of celebration, or simply putting an arm around a friend. Throughout life we need the touch of other human beings.

However, touch can be a complicated subject for adults, because of a variety of social taboos and sexual issues. Different cultures hold differing beliefs concerning acceptable levels of touch. Consequently many of us live our lives with a degree of touch starvation, although we're hardly aware of it; and the pressures of everyday life mean that most of us are used to living with ongoing tension in our bodies, which we barely notice because it feels "normal".

Touch is a powerful antidote to tension. Safe, therapeutic massage is a highly effective way to create a deep sense of relaxation and calm. It can relax and energize a tense, exhausted person, and can calm someone who is "wired" and unable to sleep.

Experiments conducted by the Touch Research Institute at the University of Miami have established many of the positive effects of touch. For example, office workers who received a short back massage through their clothes felt more alert afterward, and the level of stress hormones in their blood fell. Also, with regular massage, children with asthma had fewer attacks, and people with HIV/AIDS who were massaged daily produced more Natural Killer cells than those who weren't, and their levels of serotonin (a pain-relieving, mood-enhancing hormone) rose.

For everyone, massage is likely to lower the heart rate and blood pressure, and reduce levels of stress hormones in the body. This enables our immune system to function more efficiently and thereby helps to keep us in optimum health.

All of these extraordinary benefits spring from the simple caring touch of another human being. Massage is something that everyone can do, and this book shows you how. You will learn how to vary your touch from a gentle, relaxing stroke that releases tension, to a stronger massage that stimulates the blood circulation and lymphatic (waste disposal) system, clearing away toxins that can crystallize in the tissues and cause pain. It's good to be aware that when you massage someone, you are giving them a treatment that is both simple and powerful. There is an additional wonderful bonus: as you become more practised, you will discover that giving a massage to somebody else can make you feel relaxed and transformed – almost as though you have had a treatment yourself.

The history of massage

Massage is the most ancient form of medical care, and has been used for healing throughout recorded history. It is based on our natural human instinct to rub a sore place. Through the centuries, cultures all over the world evolved their own special styles of massage.

The earliest reference to massage is found in the *Yellow Emperor's Book of Medicine*, a Chinese book written around 2700BCE, which describes many massage techniques. Ancient Indian texts on Ayurvedic medicine, dating from around 1800BCE, also discuss massage and its benefits, as do medical texts from Egypt, Persia and Japan, dating from around 500BCE.

From Ancient Greece, Homer's epic poem the *Odyssey* (written *c.*700BCE) talks of war-weary heroes being rested and replenished with massage, and, indeed, Greek and Roman physicians used massage as a principal method of relieving pain. Hippocrates (*c.*460–*c.*377BCE), wrote that all doctors should be "experienced … in rubbing" for pain relief and relaxation.

In Ancient Rome Julius Caesar (*c.*100–44BCE) was massaged daily to relieve neuralgia. Also, the noted Greek physician Galen (129–*c.*200CE) used massage for the preparation of gladiators for combat and the treatment of injuries.

Following the decline of the Roman Empire in the 5th century, the Arabian world continued to develop the teachings and knowledge of the classical world. The philosopher and physician Avicenna (980–1037), wrote that massage could be effective "to disperse the effete matters found in the muscles and not expelled by exercise" – in effect, early sports massage.

Classical medical knowledge, including massage, re-entered Europe from the Arab world during the Renaissance of the 15th and 16th centuries. Massage was first codified as a system in Sweden, by Pehr Henrik Ling (1776–1839), forming the basis for the European styles of massage today. By the 1880s massage was increasingly popular throughout Europe and North America. Even Queen Victoria had massage, to treat rheumatic pain, lending prestige to the Swedish Massage Cure.

The first formal organization of massage practitioners in the UK, The Society of Trained Masseuses, was formed in 1894 by a group of women with nursing backgrounds. This became the Chartered Society of Physiotherapy in 1943, and gained state registration in 1966. However, later advances in medical technology and pharmacology eclipsed massage as a way for physiotherapists to work with the body.

In recent years massage has re-emerged into mainstream public awareness. There is growing appreciation of its valuable role in stress management, and it is rediscovering its place in many aspects of medicine. Modern massage is drawn from many different world traditions that share basic similarities, and it has been proved conclusively to be a safe and effective treatment.

When not to massage

Receiving regular massage is deeply beneficial for the recipient's health and well-being. However, there are a few conditions during which a person should not have massage, or should have massage only with the blessing of their medical practitioner. When you massage someone for the first time, check the following list of contraindications; these exist to protect both you and the intended recipient. If any apply to your massage partner, do not massage them until they have asked the advice of their doctor.

• Bacterial or viral infection

Do not massage someone suffering from an infectious condition as this would place additional stress on their system. Also, you could damage the affected area, and put yourself at risk from cross-infection.

• Cardiovascular conditions

Massage directly affects the circulation, so if there is an existing problem here, such as high blood pressure, angina, phlebitis, thrombosis or any coronary disease, a doctor's advice is essential.

• Fever

If someone has a fever it is unlikely they will want to be massaged. Also, it would further stress their embattled immune system.

• Pregnancy

Gentle massage is wonderful during pregnancy, but the mother-to-be should consult her midwife before any treatment.

During the first trimester the abdomen should not be massaged, and the lower back massaged only very gently (see pp.90–91).

- Severe back pain

You may be at a serious risk of exacerbating such a situation rather than improving it.

- Skin conditions

With highly infectious skin conditions, such as impetigo, avoid massage altogether. If someone has a localized fungal infection, such as ringworm or athlete's foot, or viral infection, such as verrucae, warts or herpes (cold sores), do not massage the affected area. You can massage elsewhere, but take extra care with hygiene after the massage – wash towels on a hot cycle, and clean your hands thoroughly. If the person receiving massage has any recent scar tissue, it will be fragile and tender, so avoid the area. If it feels appropriate and your friend is willing, you could simply do a gentle hold for a few moments (see p.54–55).

- Varicose veins

Massage the area with the gentlest of stroking movements or, if the veins are bad, avoid the area altogether.

Massage can be very helpful and supportive to people suffering from a variety of long-term illnesses, such as cancer, epilepsy, HIV/AIDS or psychiatric illness. However, in such cases liaison with a doctor is essential.

Understanding the body

When you give a massage, understanding a little about the body will help you to give a better treatment. The human body is nothing short of miraculous: it comprises a number of interdependent systems, including the musculo-skeletal, circulatory and nervous systems, and is exquisitely complex.

Science provides us with an increasing understanding of the links between the body systems and the mind, and explains how the activity of the body's own super-computer, the brain, has a direct impact on our physiology. A clear example of this is found in the body's stress response (or "fight-or-flight" response), whereby the brain registers a stressor or threat, and initiates a chemical cascade in the body with the intention of priming our muscles to fight or run. Physical manifestations of this include raised heart rate and blood pressure, the liver releasing more glucose into the bloodstream, and the digestive process slowing down. In a busy modern life, this response can be triggered many times a day, owing to causes ranging from work pressure, to worry about a loved one, to being stuck in traffic. Over time this undermines our immune system and makes us vulnerable to conditions such as fatigue, digestive disorders and cardiovascular illness.

Massage can bring a person's agitated physiology to a state of deeply relaxed calm. This works as the physical sensations of the massage are transmitted from the skin to the

central nervous system in the brain via
the spinal column. If stroking the skin is
experienced as a pleasant feeling, receptors
in the skin carry this message to the central
nervous system which, in turn, stimulates
relaxation in the muscles local to the
massage strokes. If these sensations continue,
a general message of relaxation will be sent
throughout the body.

WORKING WITH THE MUSCLES

There are three types of muscles in the body:
skeletal, smooth and cardiac, of which the
skeletal muscles are the ones we work on
during massage. Each muscle consists of
a bundle of contractile fibres. These are

The Skeletal Muscles of the Human Body

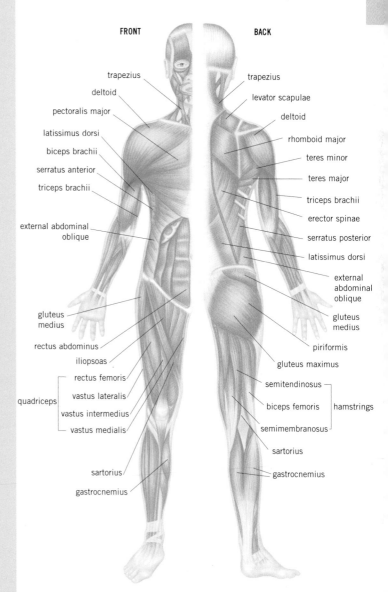

FRONT   BACK

trapezius
deltoid
pectoralis major
latissimus dorsi
biceps brachii
serratus anterior
triceps brachii
external abdominal oblique
gluteus medius
rectus abdominus
iliopsoas
rectus femoris
vastus lateralis
quadriceps
vastus intermedius
vastus medialis
sartorius
gastrocnemius

trapezius
levator scapulae
deltoid
rhomboid major
teres minor
teres major
triceps brachii
erector spinae
serratus posterior
latissimus dorsi
external abdominal oblique
gluteus medius
piriformis
gluteus maximus
semitendinosus
biceps femoris   hamstrings
semimembranosus
sartorius
gastrocnemius

enclosed in a sheath that, at each end of the muscle, extends into tendons, which are attached to bones. By contracting, muscles move our bones, giving us the power of movement. Although our skeletal muscles are under our voluntary control, we often tighten them without knowing it, leading to habitual tension being held in our bodies.

Muscles need fuel (glucose) and oxygen in order to work, and they produce metabolic waste — water, carbon dioxide and lactic acid. Lactic acid can build up in the muscles, for example after intensive exercise, irritating the nerve endings and making the muscles stiff and sore. Firm massage encourages the circulation of blood and lymph, which wash through the muscles helping to eliminate waste matter. Also, massage applied firmly in the same direction as the muscle fibres (see diagram, page 19) works on the muscle's stretch receptors, stimulating a reflex loop that sends it a message to relax.

WORKING WITH THE FLOW OF BLOOD AND LYMPH

Blood is circulated around the body via the cardiovascular system. The heart acts as a pump and sends out the blood through strong, muscular tubes called arteries to oxygenate all of our tissues. Used blood returns to the heart through veins, and the process starts all over again. Blood flows through the veins at a lower pressure than the blood in the arteries, and the veins even contain small one-way valves to stop it flowing backward. To boost the circulation of the blood, when giving massage always direct your firmer upward stroke toward the heart, with the gentler return stroke going in the opposite direction.

The lymphatic system is another circulatory system, this time moving the clear liquid lymph around the body. Lymph cleanses cells and removes toxins from them. Lymphatic ducts are found all over the body, and lymph nodes, which act as filtering stations, are situated principally in the front of the neck, the armpits and the groin. When you massage toward the heart it helps lymph move toward the nearest lymph nodes.

WORKING WITH THE ABDOMEN

The abdomen has no bony covering and contains the small and large intestines, and, in women, the reproductive organs. The small intestine is a narrow tube around 6–7m (20–23ft) in length that absorbs nutrients from digested food, and is found in the central abdominal area. The large intestine is a fatter tube around 1m (3ft) long that holds fecal material. Its three main areas – the ascending, transverse and descending colons – are situated up the left-hand side, across the top, and down the right-hand side of the abdomen respectively. It is important to massage the large intestine in a clockwise direction only, so that you are working with the natural digestive flow, and not against it.

Practical preparation

Being organized and taking care over your practical preparations is a simple but vital tool in giving a good massage treatment. Imagine receiving a massage where the masseuse's phone keeps ringing, or she runs out of oils halfway through, or you get cold and she doesn't have a blanket for you, or someone walks in unannounced – you get the picture! Good preparation also enables you to relax into giving the treatment, and this will transform the quality of your touch.

Your first task is to create a private space in which to give the massage. Choose a quiet, uncluttered room as far away from other household distractions as possible. Unless you possess a massage couch, you will need to

make a firm, padded surface on which your friend can lie. A bed is not suitable – it will be too soft, and is usually a bad height for the giver's back. One possibility is a sturdy table that stands at about your hip-height. This would need to be padded with a duvet or blankets. Alternatively you can use the floor – a futon mattress or a folded duvet covered with a large, soft towel or sheet makes a comforting texture to lie on. Whichever option you use, make sure that you can move easily all around the massage area with enough room for your legs and feet. You will also need a chair for your friend's clothes.

When you have assembled the massage area, lie down on it yourself, and check how comfortable it is. Also look at what's in your line of sight: if you are on the floor this could give you a chance to deal with any dustballs that might be lurking under cupboards!

Second, you need to consider the ambience of the room in which you are going to work. On a physical level it needs to be warm and free from draughts: many people receiving massage cool down quickly and become chilly. A quiet thermostatically-controlled blow heater can be a great help in keeping the room at an appropriate temperature. Also think about music and lighting. Keep lighting subtle and make sure no lights are shining in your massage partner's eyes when they lie down. If you (and they) would like soft music playing,

check the sound level beforehand. Make sure all phones are switched off or unplugged. A sudden loud noise can be a considerable shock to a deeply relaxed person.

Next think through the items you will need as you work. These include two clean, soft towels to cover your partner, and a light blanket in case they feel cold. A couple of pillows will also be useful – they can make a great difference to your partner's comfort. You will need a small pot of massage oil (see pp.28–29). Stand it in a bowl so that a spill is not a disaster, and place the bowl on a stable, reachable surface. It's wise to have within reach a screw-top bottle of the base oil you are using, in case you need a top-up. Keep a box of tissues handy to wipe your hands or mop up any spilled oil. You will need a clock that is clearly readable, and silent – it's easy to lose track of time when you're giving a massage. Pour yourself a glass of water in case you need a sip during the treatment (and remember to offer your partner a glass of water at the end).

The first time that somebody comes to you for a massage, you will need to run through the list of contraindications with them (see pp.16–17). It's worth making your own list, which you can photocopy, so that you have notes on file for each person you massage. If you may be giving somebody regular treatments, after the first visit make a note of how it went and which oils you used. Keep all of this information safe and secure to ensure confidentiality. If there are others in the house who may walk into the room while you are working, put a note on the door giving the time you expect to finish.

Finally, make sure that your nails are short, and that you're wearing suitable loose-fitting clothing. It's essential that you're able to move around easily, and that you don't get too hot. Tracksuit bottoms and a sleeveless or short-sleeved top are ideal.

PRACTICAL CHECKLIST

The day before:

• Make sure that your massage towels are
  clean and dry.

- Check that you have enough of your usual carrier oil to hand, and any essential oils you might be using.
- Make sure that your massage clothes are clean and ready.
- Tell others in the house that you have a massage planned and the time you have scheduled it.

An hour before:

- Lay out two folded towels, a light blanket and two pillows in your massage area.
- Make sure the room is warm enough for a person with no clothes on.
- Lay your oils out ready, including your oil pot placed in a small bowl.

- Have your contraindications checklist and a pen to hand.
- Make sure that you can see a clock.
- Check the availability and volume of music.
- Adjust lighting to the desired level.
- Put out water and two glasses.
- If necessary, place a note on the door to stop others walking in.
- Shut any pets in another part of the house.
- Have something to eat and drink.
- Change into massage clothes.

Five minutes before:

- Turn off any phones (landlines and mobiles).
- Go to the bathroom!

Managing towels

When you prepare for a massage you will need a large soft sheet or towel for your massage partner to lie on, and two towels to lay over them. There is no need to worry about getting in a tangle with the towels. It's easy.

You need towels to keep your partner warm, and to preserve their privacy. Generally you lay one towel over your partner's body, and one over their legs and hips. You could think of the towels as a "body towel" and a "legs towel".

The golden rule is: uncover only the part of the body you are about to massage. When you have finished massaging that area, replace the towel before uncovering the next part.

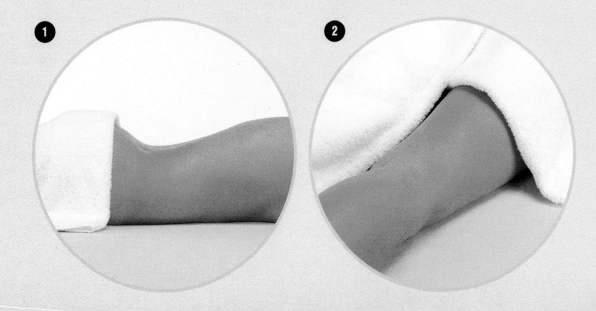

When you massage the back, either remove the body towel completely as in ①, or lay the body towel on top of the legs towel. To work on the legs, fold back enough of the relevant towel to uncover one leg; see ②. The same is true for the arms. When your partner needs to turn over, remove the legs towel completely, then hold the body towel between you and your partner, creating a screen to protect their privacy as they turn, as in ③. Finally, for massaging the abdomen, you needn't remove any towels, just fold the legs towel down to the pubic bone and fold the body towel up to the sternum, as in picture ④.

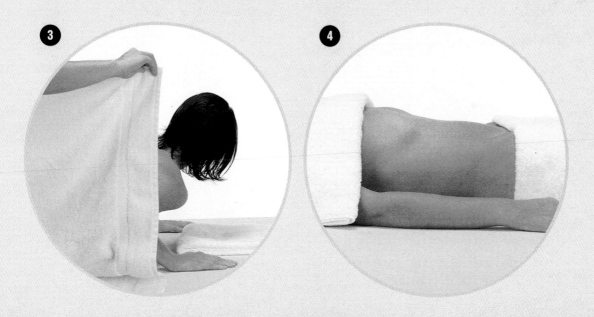

Massage oils

There is a glorious array of plant oils suitable for use in massage. We apply oil to the body so that our hands can glide, stroke or knead without pulling the skin uncomfortably. However, your choice of oil can bring additional therapeutic value to the skin.

There are two categories of oils used in massage: carrier oils (also called base oils or fixed oils) and essential oils. There are several important differences between them. The first is how they are produced. Carrier oils are extracted from plant materials, often from seeds or nuts. The best oils for massage are cold-pressed – this means that they are processed at cool temperatures, which ensures that the original therapeutic properties of the oil are not damaged or altered. Do not use commercially produced cooking oils for massage; they have been exposed to heat and chemical processing, and there is nothing therapeutic about them.

An essential oil is the distilled essence of an aromatic plant. For example, both the flowers and the leaves of lavender plants are covered in tiny sacs of aromatic oil; this is why you can rub the leaves or flowers between your fingers and smell the aroma. Most essential oil is obtained by steam distillation, whereby the aromatic compounds are released and concentrated. Very large amounts of plant material are required to make a small amount of essential oil. Always buy all of your massage oils from a specialist supplier to ensure the best possible quality.

Another basic difference between carrier and essential oils is found in their molecular structure. Carrier oils are non-volatile, which means that they don't evaporate, whereas essential oils are highly volatile; if you don't screw the lid on tightly, essential oil will evaporate quickly.

In terms of actual usage, you can apply carrier oils directly onto the skin, whereas you must always dilute essential oils with a carrier oil. As a result, carrier oils form the basis of all massage blends. They can be used alone and, indeed, have a highly nourishing and moisturizing effect on the skin. However, it is increasingly popular to use carrier oils combined with essential oils as these highly perfumed essences have a broad range of wonderful therapeutic properties to bring to a massage. Because their molecules are smaller than those of carrier oils, they are absorbed through the skin into the body where these properties act gently on the system. It is crucial, though, to follow the dilution instructions exactly – you must use only a tiny number of essential-oil drops in a much greater amount of carrier oil (see pp.128–129).

You can buy ready-made massage oils containing essential oils, or you can make your own therapeutic blends. See chapter 6, Easy Massage Oils, for more information.

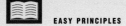
Giving massage

Once you have prepared both the room and yourself to be welcoming and ready, and have checked that there are no contraindications to massage, you're ready to give a treatment. Before you start work, make sure that you and your massage partner both know what will take place – for example, a back massage or a full-body massage – and roughly how long this will last. Say you won't talk during the massage, except to check they are comfortable.

If you sense any embarrassment about the removal of clothes the first time you give a massage to a friend or family member, be matter-of-fact. They will take their cue from you. Tell them you will go and wash your hands while they undress, and say where they should put their clothes. If they are new to massage, explain that they can either remove all of their clothes or keep on their briefs, and that their body will always be covered by towels apart from the area you are massaging. Show them where to lie down, say whether it should be on their front or back, and give them a towel to put over themselves. Go and wash your hands, and knock before you re-enter the room.

Take some time to make your partner really comfortable. If they are lying on their front, try resting their ankles and feet on a pillow (try it yourself to see how comfortable it is). If they are lying on their back, put a pillow under the backs of the knees to relax their lower back.

To begin lay relaxed hands on your partner

on top of the towel and centre yourself by taking a couple of deep breaths and relaxing your body. Take your time over this, and don't underestimate the impact it will have. Feeling your relaxed hands, and your focus on their well-being, allows your massage partner to begin the process of releasing tension.

Now, with self-awareness and relaxed breathing, focus on your partner. When you are ready, adjust the towel to uncover the area you're planning to massage. Oil your hands, put the oil pot back in its place, and begin. Check quietly from time to time that your partner is warm enough and comfortable, and if the pressure of your hands feels right. Throughout the massage it's vital to monitor your own body and breath, and to keep your body relaxed and flexible (see pp.34–35). Maintain a peaceful rhythm while you work: as you finish massaging one area of your partner's body, cover it snugly with a towel before uncovering the next area. Also use a light blanket to keep them warm.

At the end of the massage, cover your partner with the towels and blanket, and before removing your hands, mentally "end" the treatment. Some people like to silently wish their partner well. After this, pour them a glass of water, and tell them to take their time getting up and dressed. Leave the room for a few moments – you can wash your hands and stretch out your back – before returning to see how they enjoyed the experience.

Awareness of your recipient

If you have ever had the experience of receiving a massage when the masseuse seemed distracted, or worse, disinterested, you will know that this kind of massage is hardly worth having. Imagine, instead, a massage where you are treated with the greatest of care and respect, a feeling of plenty of time being taken, and a sense throughout that the masseuse, even without speaking, is fully present and focused on your well-being.

Massage is not just about knowing the right strokes to apply. Once you are past being an absolute beginner, you are ready to develop the core aspect of giving a wonderful massage – your deep awareness of the recipient as a human being. This begins with understanding that when someone places themselves in your hands for a massage, they are placing trust in you – and this trust needs to be respected.

Your awareness of the recipient of the massage applies just as much whether you give a treatment to a stranger or to a beloved one. Even with those we know well, we experience them from our own perspective, with all of the opinions and judgments that come along with this. Developing your awareness of the recipient of your massage means that, for the duration of the session, you make an inner commitment to accept them just as they are, without judgment, as another human being on their journey through life, and you care for their well-being.

Of course, this is not something you say out loud, rather it is demonstrated by your actions. Try to have everything prepared, welcoming and calm when they arrive for their massage, so you're not scampering about looking for clean towels. You want to show them that you have taken care over the whole process, and are not doing anything in a rush. Also, the first time you treat a friend, they're likely to be a bit nervous – if you are prepared and calm, it makes a big difference. When you run through the contraindications list with them, make it clear that their answers will be held in confidence. Keep the focus on your friend.

During the massage don't chat. A few people like to talk, in which case respond, but the vast majority begin to relax deeply – and in this case, chatting to them would be an invasion of their relaxation. As you massage them keep a constant inner awareness that this is another human being, with hopes and fears, joys and worries. Your job during the massage is to "guard" your friend so that they feel safe to become unguarded and, in turn, truly relaxed for the duration of the treatment. This relaxed state makes it possible for their body, mind or soul to move toward healing.

After the massage never talk to others about your partner's treatment – they may talk about it, but your job is to guard the privacy of the session, even when it's over. Always remember that giving a massage is a privilege.

Developing self-awareness

Your self-awareness during a massage is vital. It begins before the actual treatment, with good preparation (see pp.22–25). If you know that you are ready and organized, this enables you to relax and be fully aware of your partner and yourself during the massage. Throughout the treatment, try to keep about 40% of your awareness monitoring your own body and breath, and about 60% focusing on your partner. This may seem a surprising ratio, but it is highly effective. If all of your attention is on your partner, it's all too easy for your own body to become tight and exhausted without you realizing. This tension can be picked up by your partner and have a detrimental effect on the massage generally.

While you are working check frequently that your jaw is relaxed, your shoulders are dropped and your back is comfortable; and never hold your own body in one position for too long – this will strain your back and make you tired. Keep yourself moving and flexible, and always face the area on which you're working.

For anyone giving massage to family or friends, the number-one rule is to care for your own well-being and to know when you should say "no". Don't give massages if you're aware that your own energy levels are low, or if you haven't been well. Don't time massages for immediately after a full day of work, even if that would suit your friend: give yourself time for a shower and some food to replenish your energy. Care for yourself first and foremost, and your massages will a pleasure to give, and wonderfully healing for others to receive.

HOW TO RELAX YOUR BREATHING

As you read this breathe right out. This will prepare you for a deep inbreath. Now relax your stomach, and as you breathe in, gently take the breath right down to your stomach. You could imagine that this inbreath fills the whole of your body with light. Now let the breath quietly flow out; you could imagine that you are breathing out your own tension or anxiety. This forms one cycle of breath. If you can, make the outbreath longer than the inbreath: for example, breathing in, count up to four and breathing out, count to six. With practice breathing this way will help you to be centred and self-aware in any situation.

HOW TO CENTRE YOURSELF

At the start of the massage, place your hands gently on your partner on top of the towel, and take a couple of relaxed breaths. As you continue to breathe slowly and deeply, mentally scan your own body; notice where you are tense, and make an effort to relax these areas, altering your posture if it helps. Now scan your current feelings, as a compassionate observer; then put these feelings to one side. Stay aware of your breathing. Now you are ready to attend to your partner.

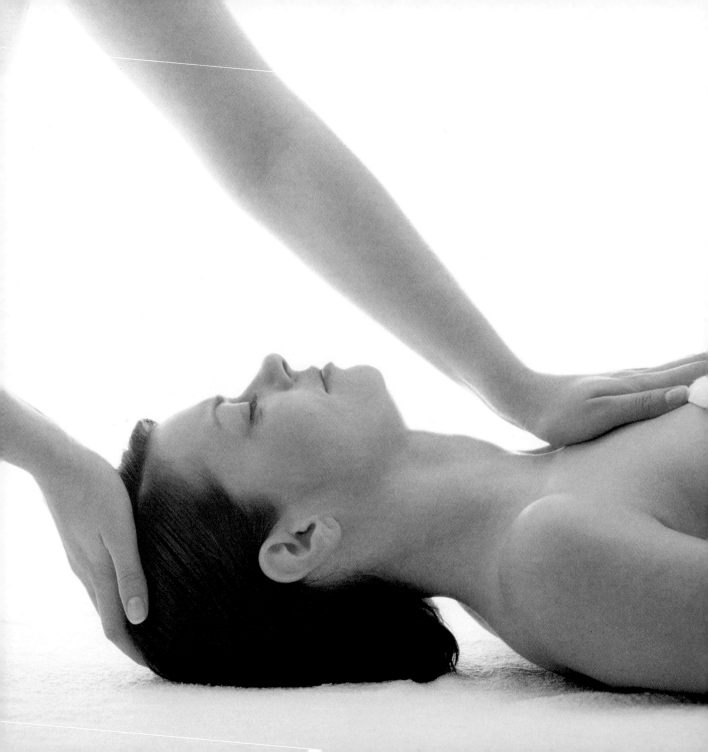

CHAPTER 2:
Easy Techniques

Your hands are an amazing piece of engineering, able to perform hundreds of different movements in daily life. They are also richly supplied with sensory nerve endings that bring you information about what you are touching. Your hands are perfectly designed, in fact, for the giving of massage.

Learning how to use your hands for massage is simple and deeply rewarding. This chapter shows you easy, basic techniques to try. I will advise you which techniques work best on different areas of the body, how a particular stroke will affect the body, and when to take special care with your choice of movements. It is well worth practising everything in this chapter many times with amenable friends, especially if you ask them for truthful feedback – in time your hands will learn which techniques you need to use, whether you are massaging someone old or young, fragile or robust.

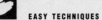

Stroking

GOOD FOR:
Beginning any massage, and for using as a connecting stroke between different techniques applied to the same, or to different, parts of the body

Stroking is the simplest, most basic touch of all. It is wonderfully calming, and all massages begin this way. Oil your hands, breathe, and relax your own shoulders and jaw. Lay your relaxed hands onto your partner, with full palm contact and your fingers together. Now smooth your relaxed palms and fingers over the contours of your partner's body as though you are gently sculpting their shape. Focus on keeping your hands relaxed, and maintain a slow, easy rhythm to your strokes. As you continue let your hands send out the message: calm.

NOTES

Stroking is used everywhere on the body, although your hands need to adapt to different body contours. The strokes are calm and flowing, ideal for beginning and ending a treatment. Stroking stretches the soft tissue, which makes it a good technique for warming an area before deeper work such as thumb circling. When working on babies, the elderly or anyone with sensitive skin, stroking may be the only technique you need (see pp.92–95 and pp.100–101). When stroking any part of the body, use gentle pressure on the upward stroke (toward the heart), and no pressure on the return stroke. This aids the circulation of blood and lymph in the body. Lymph helps to carry waste products from the muscles to the lymph nodes, and then to excrete them out of the body.

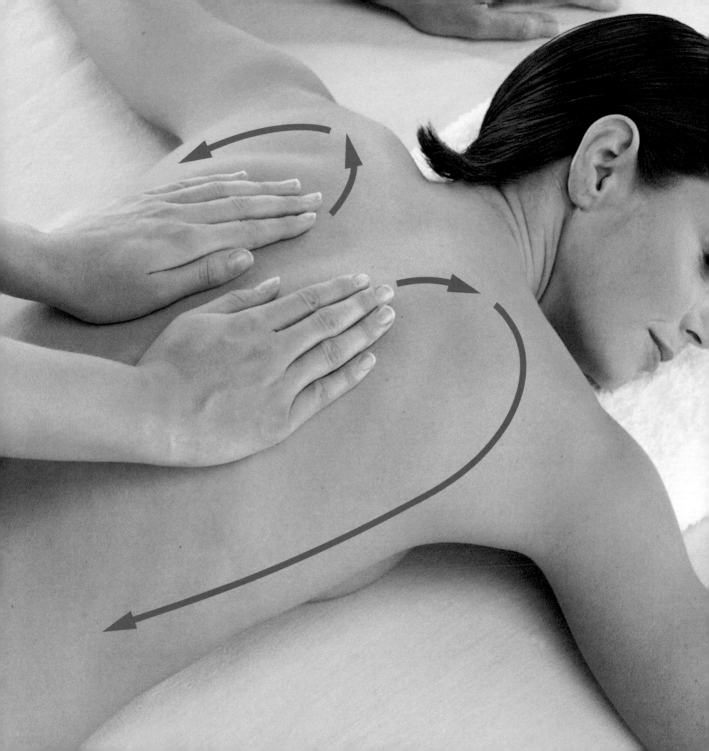

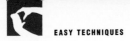
Kneading

GOOD FOR:

Warming and relaxing
tight muscles

AVOID IF:

The area you wish to
massage is affected
by varicose veins

Kneading is a rhythmic stroke that warms and relaxes the soft tissue. It is used on the back and shoulders, and on fleshy areas such as the buttocks, thighs and calves. The movement is like kneading dough. Place your hands flat on the body, with your elbows apart. With your right hand, pick up the flesh and in one fluid movement, gently squeeze it and release it into your other hand. With your left hand, gently squeeze the flesh and release back into the right hand. Continue with this rhythmic movement, moving forward and back over the area you are massaging until it feels warm and pliable.

NOTES

You can use kneading as a soothing stroke as it is repetitive and gentle. It will both relax your partner and warm the area you are massaging. It can also be applied more vigorously. This can be useful when you are working on muscles that are tired or aching, following exertion. Deep kneading will not only soften the tissues but will also boost the circulation in the area you are working on. This in turn speeds up the elimination of metabolic waste and helps the muscles to recover from exercise (see pp.96–97).

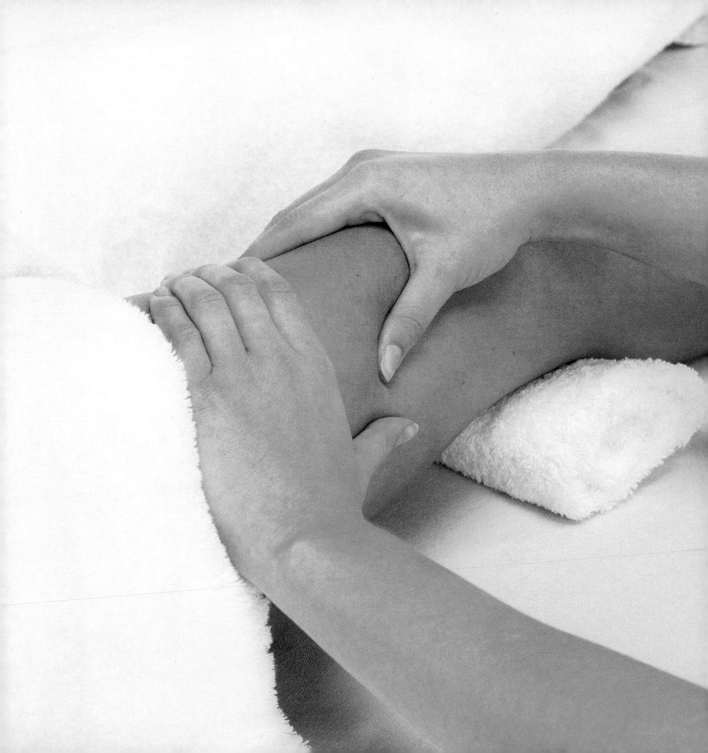

Thumb circling

GOOD FOR:
Loosening deep, chronic muscle tension

TAKE CARE IF:
Muscles are tight and tender – keep checking that the pressure feels good to your partner

AVOID IF:
The area you wish to massage is affected by varicose veins

Thumb circling is a technique whereby you use your thumbs to work firmly into the muscles. Place the pads of your thumbs on the skin and lean into them. Make small, penetrating circles into the muscle. Then glide your thumbs to the next area and repeat the circles. This helps to release deep, habitual muscular tension. It also helps to disperse the toxins that are the metabolical byproducts of muscle use. You can apply thumb circling wherever you feel small nodules of tension, or granular deposits in the tissues. It feels wonderful if you work your way up the muscles on either side of your massage partner's spine.

NOTES

Thumb circling requires an increased level of pressure, so before you use it, make sure you take time to warm the area you are working on, using stroking or kneading techniques. If you apply thumb circling too soon or too deep, it will cause discomfort, which is counterproductive. So stroke or knead the area first, until it feels warm under your hands. When you move on to thumb circling, sink your thumbs into the tissues gently at first, gradually increasing the pressure; and check with your partner that this increased pressure feels comfortable.

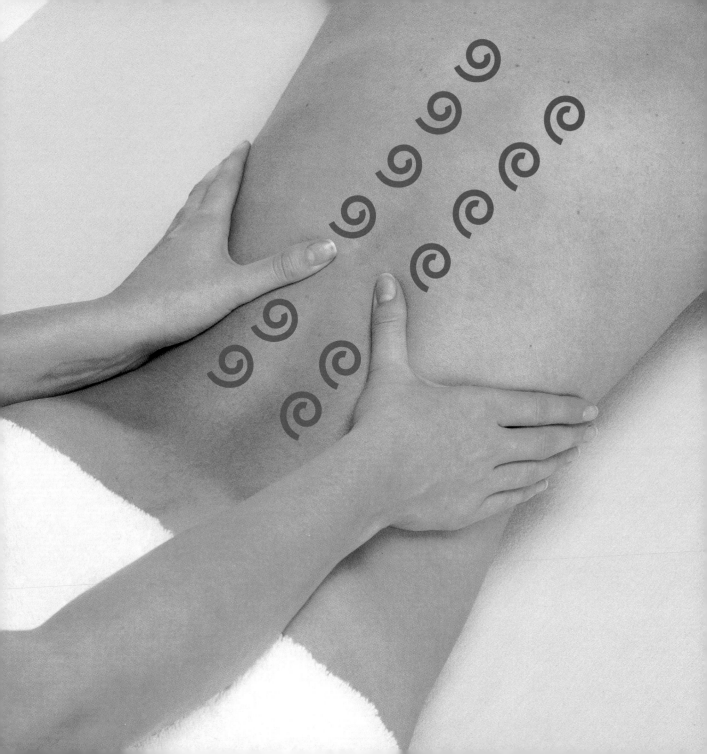

Knuckling

GOOD FOR:
Unknitting and relaxing tense muscles, and for stimulating the circulation

TAKE CARE IF:
The skin is delicate, or if you're massaging a very thin person

AVOID IF:
The area you are massaging has any varicose veins

Knuckling can be a highly satisfying stroke to receive. Curl your hands into loose fists and lay the middle section of your fingers on the skin. Now lean through your hands and rotate your knuckles in small, circular movements. If you prefer you can knuckle with one hand, using your other hand for support. You can vary the pressure by leaning into your hands with more or less of your body weight. This stroke feels great on the back, buttocks, palms of the hands and soles of the feet. You can work quite deeply without the pressure feeling uncomfortable, but take care not to knuckle across bone.

NOTES

You can also try a technique known as "straight" knuckling, where you keep your knuckles flat on the skin and simply push them firmly along the surface rather than rotate them.

For example, when working up the thighs, you can lean into your hands and glide your knuckles firmly up the thigh in the direction of the heart (see pp.20–21). This form of

knuckling works quite deeply into the body's tissues, so it is particularly useful for areas suffering from chronic tension or where the tissues feel congested.

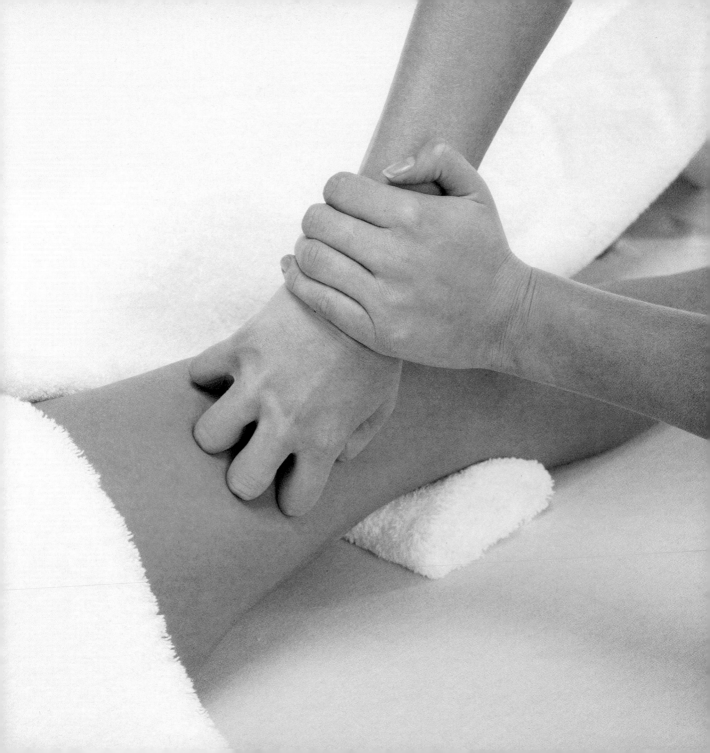

Pulling

GOOD FOR:
Working on the sides of the body where it can be difficult to apply other techniques

Pulling is a kind of stroking, using the whole of your palm and fingers, usually pulling upward on the sides of the body. Instead of leaning your weight forward into the stroke, you use your weight to pull toward yourself. For example, working from one side of your partner's abdomen, lean forward and wrap your palm and fingers around the top of their hip on the far side, then lean back, pulling your hand toward you — follow straight on with your other hand. By alternating your hands you can work your way up the side of the abdomen.

NOTES

When you have pulled all the way along your partner's opposite side, and you want to work on the side closest to you, simply move round to the opposite side of their body. Alternatively, you can stay where you are and make the movement a push instead of a pull, stroking alternate hands up from their nearside hip and across the abdomen.

You can try another wonderful pull when your partner is lying on their front. Position yourself at their head, lay your hands flat on their shoulders with fingers pointing toward their hips and stroke down either side of the spine; when you reach the hips, separate your hands so they glide out to the sides of the hips and then leaning back, pull slowly and firmly up your partner's sides with both hands.

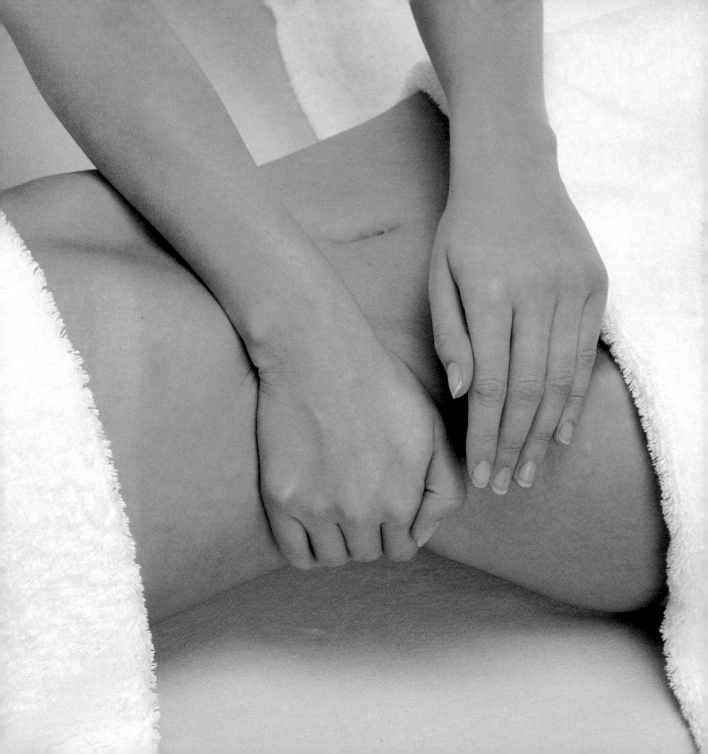

Whole-hand frictions

GOOD FOR:
Warming an area that feels cold and tight

TAKE CARE IF:
The skin is fragile or delicate

Lay both your hands on your partner, with full palm contact and fingers relaxed and close together. Now, without applying much pressure, rub your hands vigorously forward and back in opposite directions. This friction generates a healthy heat in the skin. Rub over one area until you feel the heat building – you will sometimes see the area becoming pink – then, without stopping the frictions, move your hands to the next area, and continue until you feel the tissues are warm and enlivened. If you find your hands getting tired, relax them more without slowing down. Rubbing for a minute or so should be enough to warm each area.

NOTES

Whole-hand frictions are useful from time to time when you find you are working on an area of the body that not only feels chronically tense but also chilly. Areas of tension should always be warmed, normally using stroking and kneading, before you begin any deeper strokes. Once in a while you may find that despite your best efforts, the tissues seem to stay cold and unyielding. Check that the room is warm and that your partner actually feels warm enough; if they seem fine then try whole-hand frictions to warm the cold area.

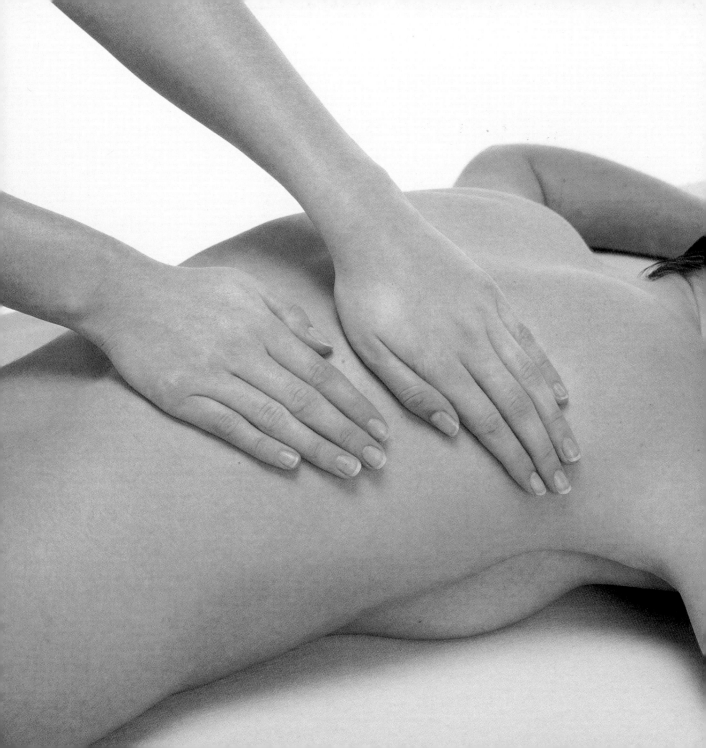

Hacking

✓ GOOD FOR:
Boosting the local
circulation in an area
of the body

✗ AVOID IF:
The area on which you
want to work is bony,
or if it has varicose
veins or sensitive skin

Hacking is an invigorating stroke, which you can use to stimulate the circulation in the muscles. Keeping your arms and wrists completely relaxed, use the outer sides of your hands alternately to strike up and down on your partner's shoulders, buttocks or thighs. This is a fast move, and it works best if you have the palms of your hands quite close to one another, so your fingers brush rapidly past each other as you move. If you allow your arms and wrists to become tense, hacking can start to feel like karate chopping, so keep checking that they are relaxed all the time you are applying this technique.

NOTES

If you would like to try some hacking on your massage partner, be sure to warm the area with stroking and kneading first. Use hacking only on fleshy areas, such as the buttocks or thighs, or on the shoulders if they are very muscular. It is a stroke that leaves the skin warm and glowing. Don't use hacking on bony areas, sensitive skin or near varicose veins as this could damage them or cause discomfort. Also, don't use hacking on your partner if you are aiming to give them a wholly tranquil treatment or if they have fallen asleep.

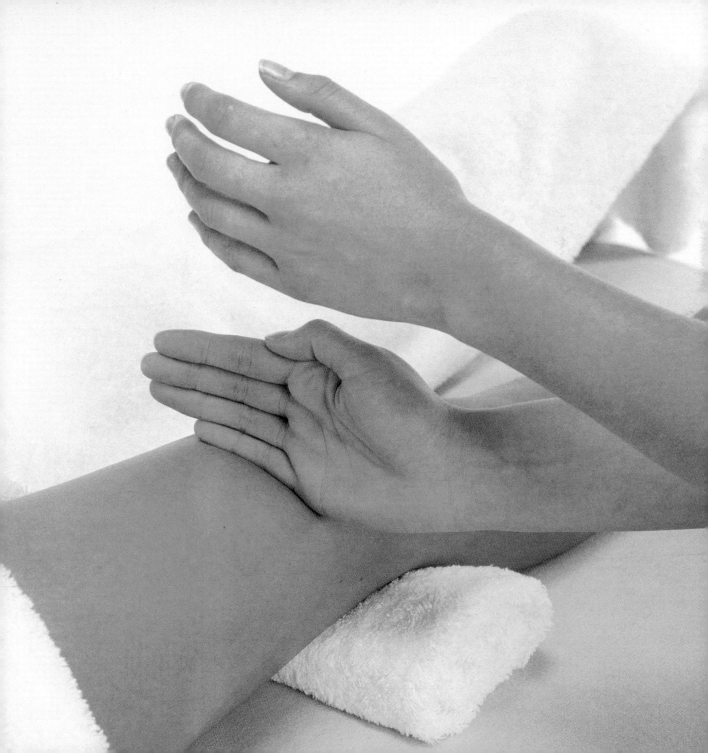

Stretching

 GOOD FOR:

Giving a sense of
elongated relaxation
to a tight back

Place your forearms side by side across the centre of your partner's back, then slowly move your forearms apart, with constant gentle pressure. Keep going until one forearm is over your partner's sacrum (at the very base of the spine) and the other just below the base of their neck. This stretch feels wonderful to receive. You can also try it using your hands. Don't press hard directly on the vertebrae: keep gentle pressure across the whole of your palms. Imagine that you are gently elongating the spine. At the end of the stretch, let one hand rest on the sacrum and the other just below the neck for a few moments.

NOTES

Gentle passive stretches can ease chronic contraction in the body, reminding it how it can elongate and relax. Stretches are most effective when they are applied toward the end of working on an area of the body. Imagine trying to stretch a piece of cold, tight modelling clay: it's much easier when you've warmed it and worked it first. People love to receive the forearm stretch at the end of a back massage — repeat it several times. Also, you can synchronize with your partner's breath, beginning the stretch on their outbreath.

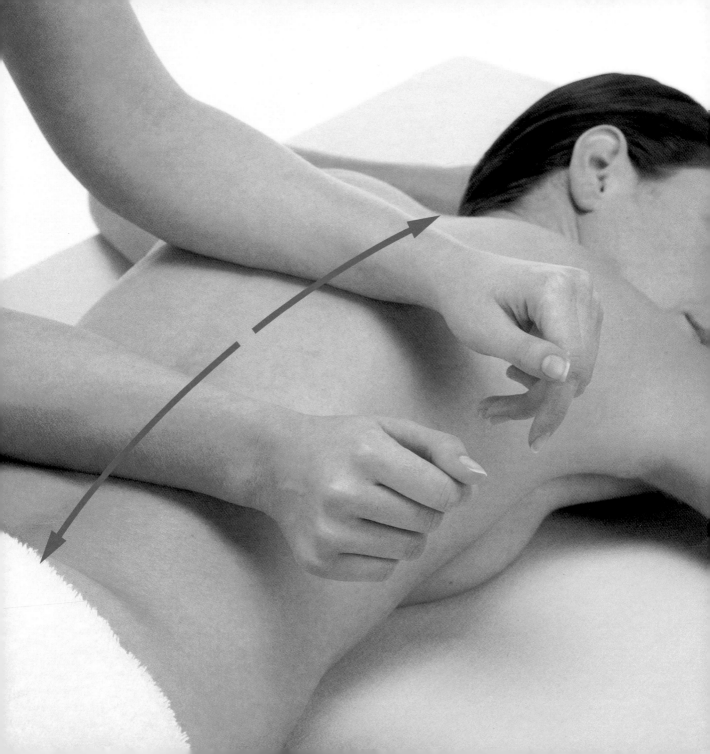

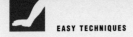

Simple holding

GOOD FOR:
Beginning and ending a massage – it creates focus and calm in the giver, and a sense of safety in the receiver of the treatment

Holding means simply laying your hands on your partner and focusing your care and respect for them by doing so. This kind of simple hold feels deeply relaxing, comforting and nurturing to receive, and it is calming for you as well as your partner. You can lay your hands in a simple hold on your partner's back, abdomen, or upper chest and head. Don't lean on your hands, or apply any pressure with them; rather make your touch a conscious "laying-on of hands" that provides a meditative moment in your session. Allow your breathing to deepen, and the rest of the world to fall away. Take your time.

NOTES

You can begin your massage session with a simple hold, which will focus you, and settle your massage partner into receiving a healing process. Maintain it for a minute or two, remembering not to apply any pressure; this touch will make your partner feel safe and relaxed. Put your awareness into your palms: they will sometimes feel alive and tingling. You can end the massage this way too, and send your silent blessing to your partner before removing your hands if you wish. Let yourself enjoy this hold too: it is very special.

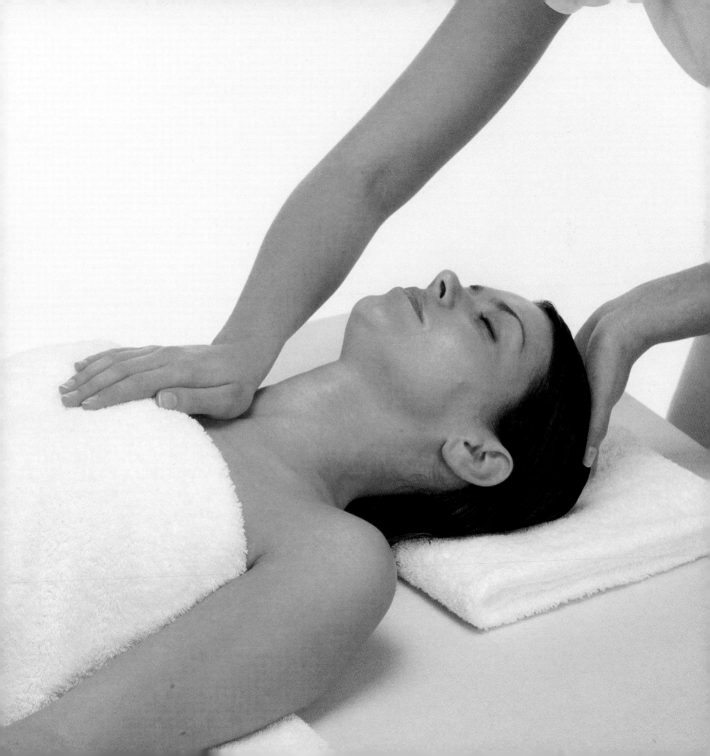

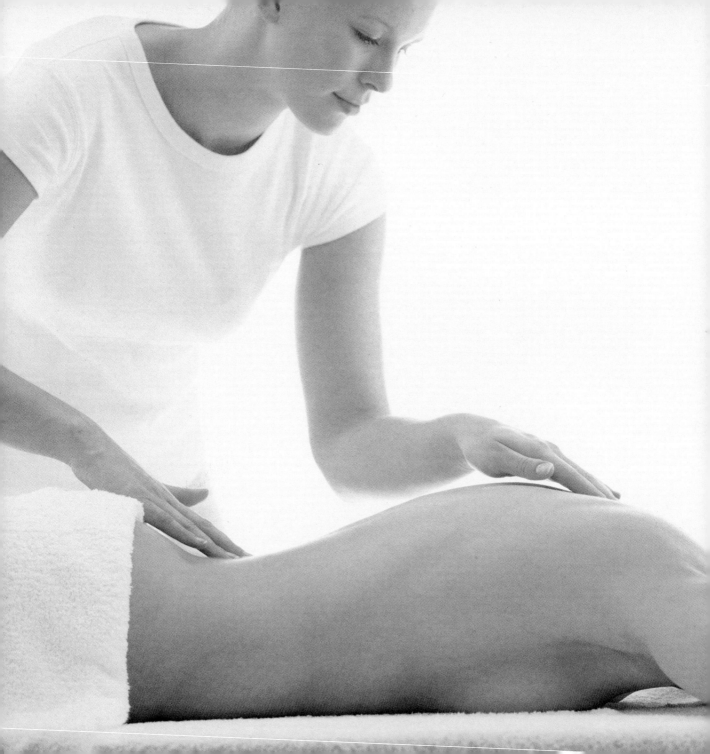

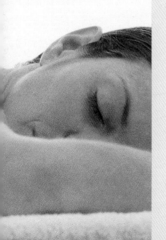

CHAPTER 3:
Easy Routines

O nce you feel at ease with the basic techniques of massage, it's time to link these techniques together to create a massage routine. In this chapter I will take you through a short routine for the shoulders and neck (pp.58–59), and then seven further routines for other parts of the body. These can either be performed individually, or can be linked together to form a wonderful full-body routine. A good routine begins with you relaxing and warming your massage partner's muscles, then adapting your movements to whatever best suits the recipient. Be aware that no massage routine is written in stone; as you gather experience you will want to exercise more flexibility within a treatment session. For example, you might want to spend longer working on particularly tense shoulders. However, even massage professionals keep the basics of a routine in mind, like a simple road map to keep you on track.

The shoulders and neck

This short treatment can transform someone who has had a bad day at work. You will need two chairs. Wrap a towel around your partner's torso, and seat them comfortably. Sit behind them, oil your hands, centre yourself and make contact with their upper back. ① With hands flat, begin stroking the area between the shoulder blades, then work up to the neck, out over the shoulders and back to where you began. Keep your fingers relaxed and your palms in full contact with the skin. ② When the area is warm, place your thumbs either side of the spine just below neck level. Begin thumb-circling, drawing small circles with your

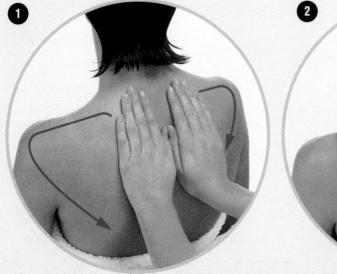

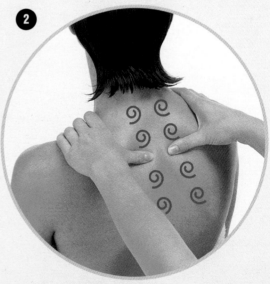

thumbs and leaning into them. Work down to towel level then back up to the neck.

③ Keeping contact, stand at your partner's side, facing their right shoulder. Gently squeeze the back of the neck several times, using your fingers and thumb to press under the base of the skull. ④ Holding the shoulder between your hands, apply more thumb-circling with alternate thumbs, working along the top of the shoulder to the neck. Repeat this on the other shoulder. Moving behind your partner again, repeat the upper back stroking in ①.

Finish by sweeping your fingertips several times out from the neck and off the shoulders.

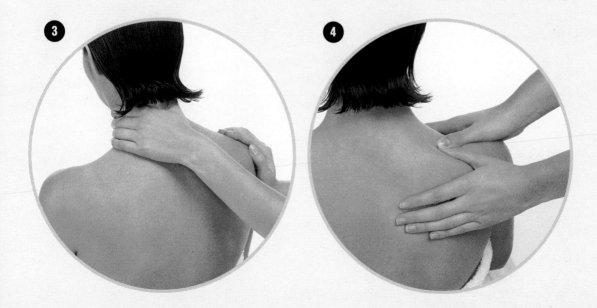

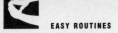
The back

Make your partner comfortable lying on their front. Lay one towel over their legs and hips and another over their back. When you're ready to begin, remove the back towel and fold the other towel down so that you can massage the entire back. Spread your massage oil with smooth strokes over the area.

① Position yourself at your partner's head, and relax your hands onto their shoulders. Leaning into your hands, stroke down both sides of the spine to below the waist. Separate the hands and slide them out to hold each side of the hips. Lean your weight backward, so your hands slide up the sides to below the

1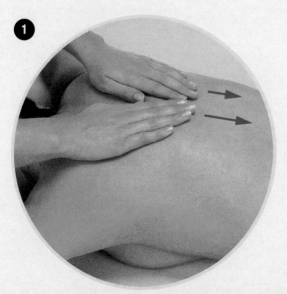

2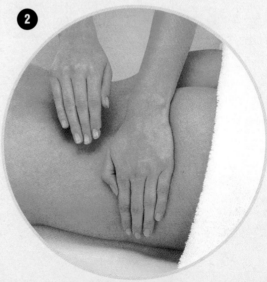

armpits, giving your partner a good stretch. Repeat several times. ② Keeping contact, move to your partner's side. Starting at hip level, wrap one hand around their opposite hip and gently pull, sliding your hand toward the spine. Alternate your hands and work your way up from hip to armpit level. Repeat on the side closest to you, this time pushing rather than pulling. ③ Place your hands one on top of the other over the sacrum, and make gentle, slow circles over the sacral area, until it feels warm. ④ Now stroke up the back, separate the hands out over the shoulders, and stroke back down to the sacrum. Repeat several times.

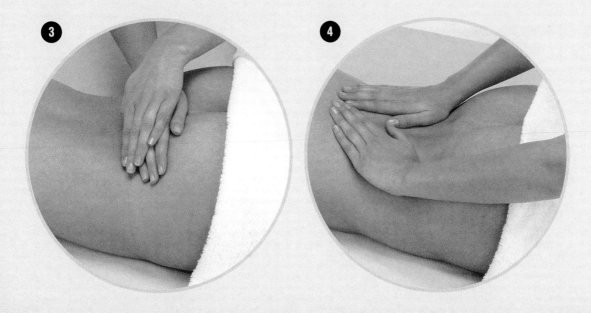

⑤ Begin kneading the buttock on the far side. Pick up the flesh squeezing gently with your whole hand, and release it into your other hand. Make sure you use the whole hand so you don't pinch. Knead rhythmically from one hand to the other until the area is warmer and less tense. ⑥ Now knuckle the buttock, using one hand; relax your other hand onto the sacrum. You can knuckle quite firmly, but don't knuckle the bone at the upper edge of the pelvis. ⑦ Now, using the muscle at the base of your thumb, "drain" the area you have knuckled, smoothing firmly out over the buttock. Move to your partner's other side

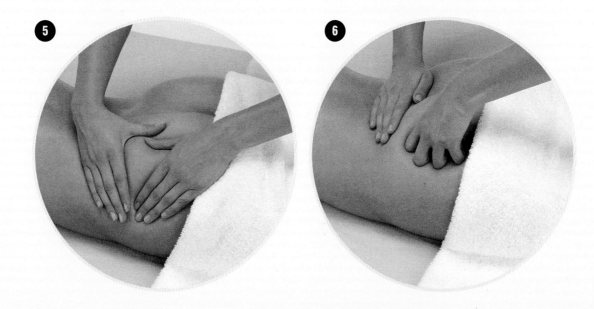

and repeat the kneading, knuckling and draining, on the other buttock. Stroke the entire back again several times, as in step ④: each time you work on one smaller area, use this unifying stroke to reconnect the whole back. ⑧ Position your thumbs each side of the spine, just above the sacrum, fingers out to the sides. Begin thumb circling, working your way up the sides of the spine, all the way to the base of the neck. Some people's backs are tense and tender in particular areas; ask your partner if they would like more pressure or less as you work. Stay a little longer on the tight areas. Repeat several times.

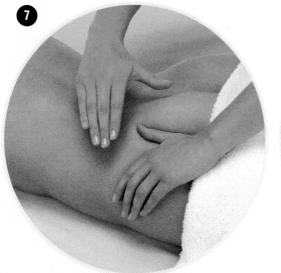

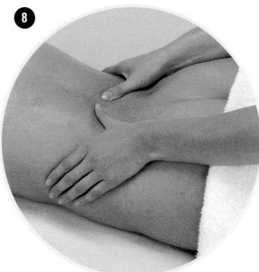

⑨ Still thumb circling, work your thumbs over the area between the spine and shoulder blades, moving the thumbs gradually up to the shoulders. Work your way across the tops of the shoulders, then return to stroking the entire back again. ⑩ Still standing at your partner's side, turn to face their back. Lean forward and lay your forearms side by side across the middle of the back; now slowly, with pressure, move your forearms apart until one forearm is down at the sacrum, the other at the base of the neck. This is a wonderful stretch; repeat it several times. ⑪ Next, with one hand, position your forefinger and tallest

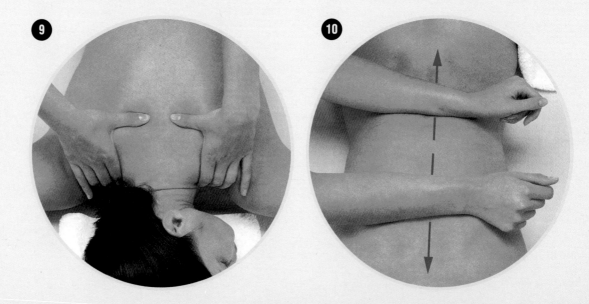

finger one each side of the spine at the base of the neck. Lay your free hand on the back of your working hand for support. Now, with pressure, pull your fingers down either side of the spine to the sacrum. Stroke the entire back again. ⑫ Finish with a simple hold, relaxing one hand onto the sacrum and the other on the upper back. Stay like this for a few moments. You can send your silent blessing to your partner if you wish. When you have finished, lay the towel over your partner's back again. If the treatment is finishing here, give them a few moments of peace, before helping them up and giving them a glass of water.

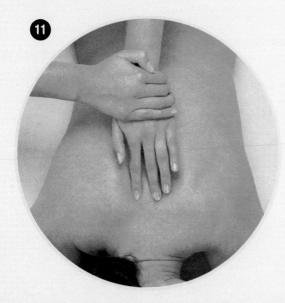

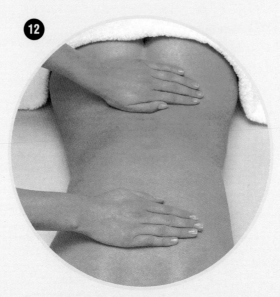

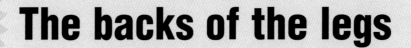

The backs of the legs

This simple routine is designed to follow the back massage, as part of a whole-body routine. Your partner may like to have their ankles and feet laid on a towel or pillow. Lay one towel over the body, and another over the legs and hips. When you are ready, fold the leg towel back diagonally, so one leg is visible but the hips are still covered. Oil the leg with smooth strokes. ① Lay your hands on the back of the ankle, palms next to each other and your fingers pointing in opposite directions. Drape your fingers so they enclose the leg on both sides. Leaning slightly through your hands, stroke them upward toward the buttock.

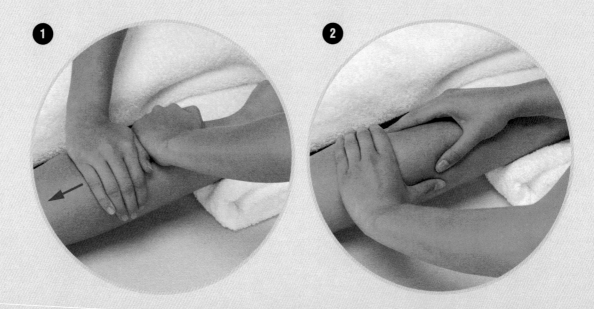

Separate the hands, draw them down the sides of the leg and down over the sole of the foot. Repeat this stroke several times. ② Moving round to the side of the leg, knead the calf muscle until it feels relaxed and warm. ③ Now knead your way up the back of the thigh in the same way. ④ Slip your hand under your partner's ankle and raise it, until their calf is at right-angles to the thigh. Support the ankle with one hand, and with the other stroke firmly down from ankle to back of the knee several times. Lay the leg down. Repeat step ①, stroking up the whole leg. Replace the towel and repeat the routine on the other leg.

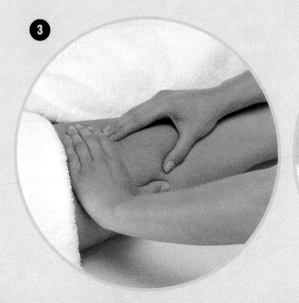

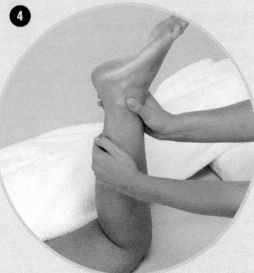

The fronts of the legs

This routine usually forms part of a whole-body massage. Help your partner to turn onto their back. Most people find it blissfully comfortable to have a pillow under the backs of the knees. You might like to try out the position to see for yourself. Your partner will need a towel over their body and another over their legs. When you are ready to begin, fold the leg towel back diagonally so that the leg is visible but the hips are covered. Spread your massage oil with smooth strokes over the whole area, including the foot, which you should sandwich between both of your hands. ① Lay your hands on the front of the ankle, with your palms next each other and your fingers pointing in opposite directions. With full palm contact and fingers draped around the leg, lean into your hands and stroke them up the leg. Take the pressure off as you go over the knee. Continue up the thigh, then separate your hands and draw them down the sides of the legs all the way to the foot. Sandwich the foot, one hand on top, one hand on the sole,

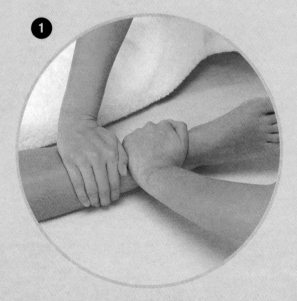

and draw your hands off at the toes. Repeat this entire move several times. ② Without losing contact, position yourself beside the thigh and begin kneading firmly, working on the front of the thigh and the outer thigh; be sensitive about your partner's privacy and don't knead the inner thigh. ③ With one hand knuckle over the area you have just kneaded. Hold the wrist of your knuckling hand with your other hand for support. Check with your partner that the pressure feels right. The tissues of the thighs can be sluggish in some people – this move stimulates the circulation, encouraging the excretion of toxins.

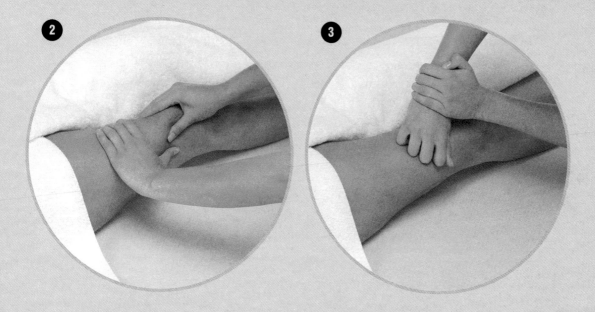

④ Now, making a V-shaped space between your fingers and thumbs on both hands, stroke firmly up the thigh, alternating the hands so one follows the other. ⑤ Without losing contact, move next to your partner's calf. Wrap your hands around and under the knee so that it is supported but your thumbs are free. Beginning at the top of the knee, apply slow thumb circling, right around the edge of the kneecap, to a depth that feels comfortable to your partner. Now use your fingers to massage gently under the back of the knee. ⑥ Make a V-shaped space between your finger and thumb as before, but this time lay

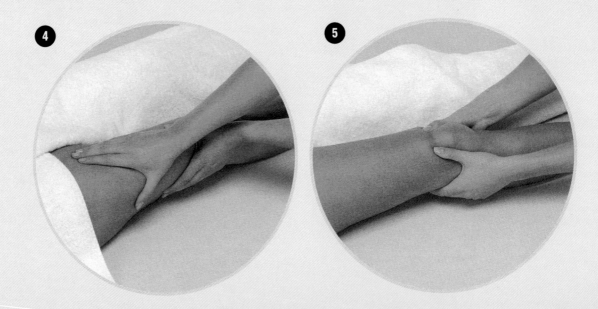

one hand over the other so that the two Vs are exactly one on top of the other. Position this V just below your partner's knee, then wrap your fingers around the leg. Now push your hands up the leg, taking your weight off as you go over the knee, and push past the knee a short way. Repeat this several times. ⑦ Now cradle the ankle between your palms using the muscles at the base of your thumbs to circle several times around the ankle bones. Finish by repeating step ①, stroking up the leg from ankle to thigh and back down again, finally sandwiching the foot between both hands. Now repeat all steps on the other leg.

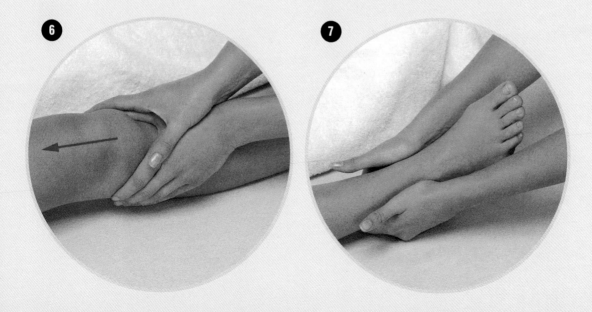

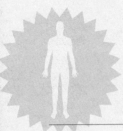

The feet

Massaging the feet is a highly effective way of relaxing the whole body. If your partner is lying down, you can tuck a pillow under their knees; if sitting, ensure they are comfortable and relaxed, with their legs supported on a stool. Lay a towel underneath the legs, and have another towel to hand. Begin by oiling the lower legs and feet with smooth movements, sandwiching the feet between your hands. Then cover one leg and foot with the second towel. ① Lay your hands on the front of your partner's ankle, with your palms next to each other and fingers pointing in opposite directions. Drape your fingers around the leg, so that you are holding it on both sides. Leaning your weight gently through

your hands, stroke them up toward the knee. Stop before the knee, separate the hands and draw them back down the sides of the leg to the ankle. Now slide one hand under the back of the heel and the other on the top of the foot; sandwich the foot, and draw your hands up to the toes and off the ends. Repeat this

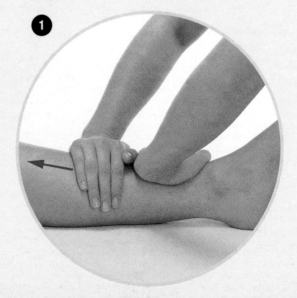

move several times. ② Now clasp both of your hands around the foot, with your thumbs on the sole under the arch, and your fingers tightly over the top. Squeeze firmly, and maintaining this level of pressure, slide up to the toes and off. If your partner likes this move (most people do), you can repeat it several times. ③ Next, lay one hand flat on top of the foot, and use your other hand to knuckle all over the sole in tiny circles. You can knuckle quite firmly working over the ball, arch and heel of the foot. Even people with ticklish feet usually enjoy this move, as it is deep and firm.

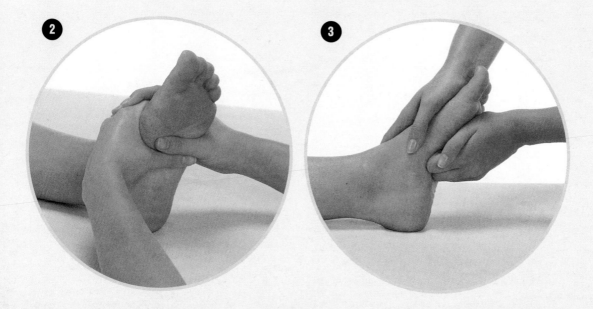

④ Now open out your knuckling hand and use it to support the sole of the foot with full palm contact. With your other hand, stroke firmly from the base of the toes up to the ankle, several times. ⑤ Now slide your hands one each side of the foot so that your fingers are lying on the ankle bones. Use your fingertips to massage around the ankle bones, working in tiny circles. This movement feels best if you work quite firmly. The ankle is a hard-working, complex joint, so give it lots of attention. ⑥ Now slide one hand underneath the heel to support it, and slide your other hand about a hand's width up the back of the calf; take hold

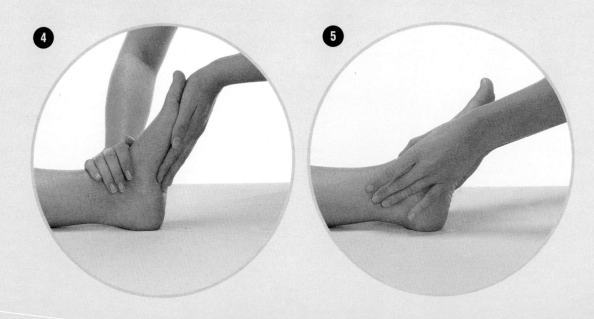

of the Achilles tendon between thumb and the side of your forefinger, and gently pull your hand down to the heel. Alternate your hands, so one supports the heel and the other pulls down the tendon. Do this several times. ⑦ Next, steady the foot with one hand, and use the other hand to massage each of the toes in turn, squeezing and then pulling gently as though lengthening them. Finish by repeating step ①, stroking from foot to knee and back again with both hands, and finally sandwich the foot between your hands for a few moments before removing them. Cover the foot with a towel and repeat all moves on the other foot.

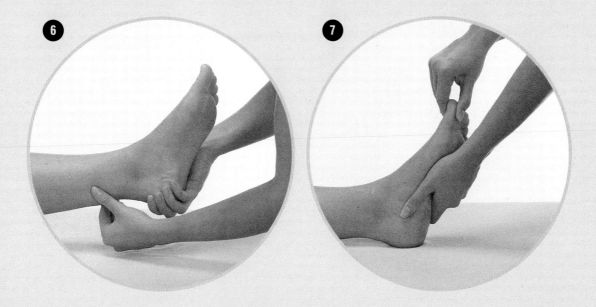

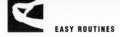

The abdomen

You should perform this routine as part of a whole-body massage. Take particular care when massaging the abdomen because it holds vital digestive organs that are unprotected by bony structure. Uncover the abdomen from the sternum to just above the pubic bone. Spread your massage oil over the area gently.

① Lay your hands flat on the abdomen in a "fir tree" shape, fingers pointing toward the chest, and your partner's navel appearing in the window between your thumbs. Slide your hands up to the sternum then back down again, and when the navel appears through the thumb "window", separate your hands and, fingers

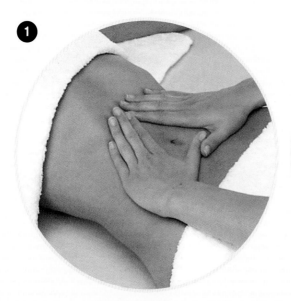

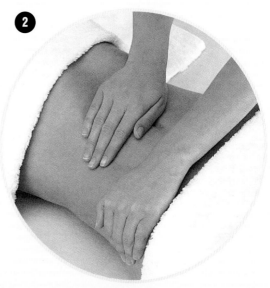

first, slide them under the back on either side of the body. Lift very slightly, then pull the hands back round to the front, and repeat several times. ② Wrap your left hand around your partner's right hip; pull up gently and, using alternate hands, pull along the side from hip to upper towel level. Do the same on the side closest to you, this time pushing rather than pulling. ③ Crossing over your hands, apply small strokes with alternate hands around the abdomen, moving in a clockwise direction. ④ With hands one on the other, slowly circle them around the navel several times, and finish with them resting below the navel.

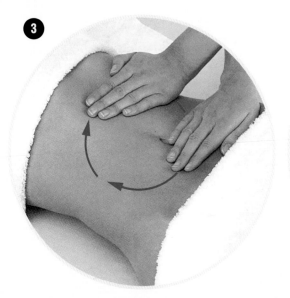

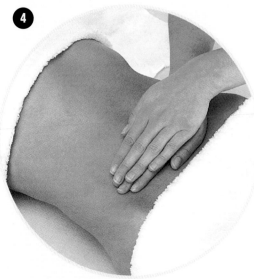

The arms and hands

This routine usually forms part of a whole-body massage. Alternatively, you could also start at step ④ to give a simple hand massage, which is a highly soothing and relaxing treatment to receive in itself. If you are performing this routine as part of a whole-body massage, where your partner has towels covering their body, simply uncover one arm; if they are sitting up, support their lower arm and hand on the arm of a chair, with a towel underneath. Encourage your partner to relax the arm and hand completely, like a rag doll. Oil the hand, arm and shoulder with smooth strokes. ① Take your partner's right hand in your own right hand. Hold their hand in a supportive and comfortable clasp and lay your other hand on the back of the wrist, with the outer edge of your hand facing up toward the elbow. Now stroke with that hand all the way up the arm, round the top of the shoulder and return down the back of the arm. End by sandwiching their hand between both of your hands. Repeat this move several times.

1

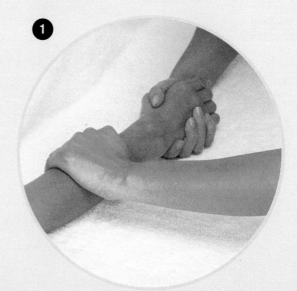

② Still holding the hand, use your free hand to take the wrist between your thumb and fingers; keeping a firm hold, slide your hand up toward the elbow, squeezing the forearm gently as you go, and bring your hand back down to the wrist. Repeat this move several times, moving your grip slightly each time.

③ Ease your right hand out of your partner's hand, and slide it under the inside of their elbow, holding it steady, so that their forearm lies on top of, or alongside, your own. With your other hand, gently knead your way up their upper arm and around the top and back of their shoulder.

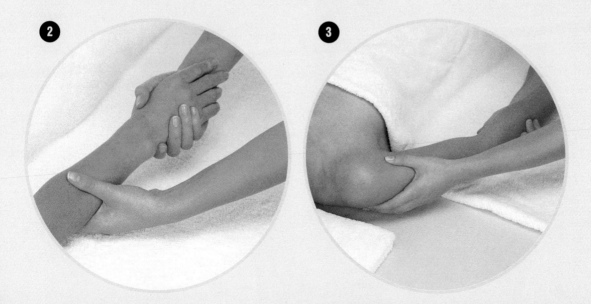

If you want to work on the hands alone, this is the place to begin (with oiled hands). Sandwich your partner's hands between yours for a moment. ④ Wrap your hands under their wrist, so that your thumbs are free to do tiny circles on the back of their wrist: explore the bones of the wrist with your thumbs.

Supporting your partner's elbow and hand, gently turn the forearm over, and repeat the tiny circles on the inside of their wrist.

⑤ Slide one hand to support underneath your partner's upturned palm, and use the base of the thumb on your other hand to circle, slowly and firmly, around their palm. You can also

4

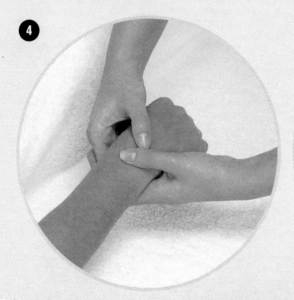

5

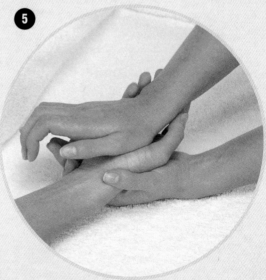

gently knuckle the palm, moving your knuckles in small circles. ⑥ Gently turn the hand back over so the back of the hand is uppermost. Supporting the palm with your fingers, use your thumbs to stroke from the base of the fingers to the wrist. Do this with alternate thumbs. ⑦ Now supporting your partner's hand with one hand, use your free hand to massage the thumb and each finger from base to tip, pulling and squeezing gently up the length of each digit and off the end. End by sandwiching your partner's hand between your hands for a few moments, before slowly drawing your hands away. Repeat all the moves on the other arm and hand.

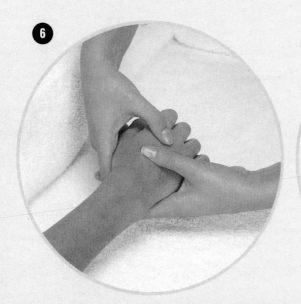

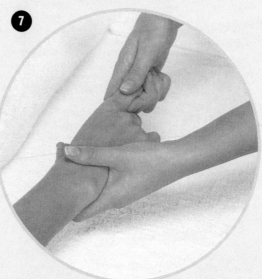

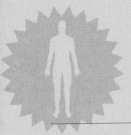

The shoulders, face and head

This heavenly treatment can be a complete session in itself, or can form the final part of a full-body massage. Having your face touched is a surprisingly intimate experience for most people, so your touch needs to be both tender and respectful. Your partner should be lying on their back, with a pillow under their knees and towels over their upper body and legs. If your partner has long hair, spread it upward, away from the neck. Fold the top towel down to uncover the upper chest and spread oil over this area and around the shoulders, with smooth strokes. ① Position yourself behind your partner's head. Lay your hands side by side on their upper chest and stroke them out to the shoulders, and round and under the shoulders until they meet under the back of the neck. If the last part seems difficult, try this: as your hands stroke under the backs of the shoulders, press the backs of your hands down into the towel your partner is lying on. This can help you to get under the shoulders. Even if it feels awkward to you, it is likely to

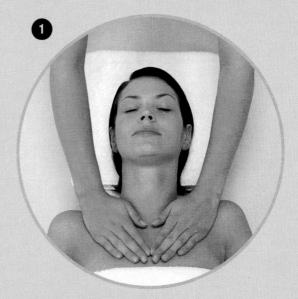

❶

feel good to your partner. Repeat this stroking movement several times. ② Now knuckle across the chest, remembering to be very gentle where you can feel the collar bones. Knuckle more firmly out around the shoulders and underneath to the back of the neck. Then repeat step ①, stroking the whole area. Now oil the neck and face with gentle strokes, touching only lightly on the front of the throat. ③ Using alternate hands sweep lightly from your partner's collarbone up to their jaw bone, starting at the left side and working round to the right. As you move on to massaging the face, keep your hands very relaxed, but not

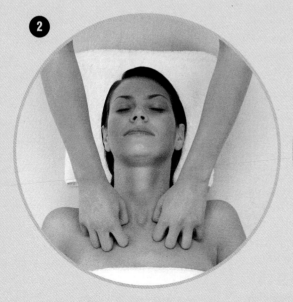

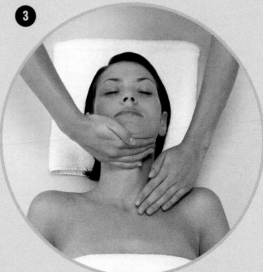

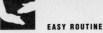

tentative. Your touch needs to be both tender and confident; keep the pace very peaceful. For your partner, having the face that they present to the world touched in this way can be profoundly relaxing. ④ Cup your partner's chin with one hand, then sweep this same hand gently up one side of their face. As you do this cup the chin with the other hand and then sweep this hand up the other side of their face. Do this stroke, alternating your hands, several times. Always remember to keep your hands relaxed and tender. ⑤ Now lean slightly to your right, and sweep with alternate hands up the right side of your partner's face

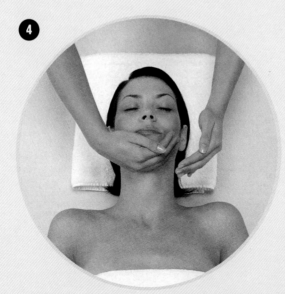

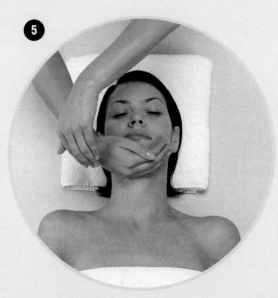

several times. Then lean to your left, and repeat the move, this time sweeping up the left side of the face. ⑥ Next, with the flats of your fingers, stroke your partner's nose from the tip to the bridge with alternate hands. Repeat this several times. ⑦ Now lay one hand sideways across your partner's forehead, fingers pointing to their temple. Stroke gently across the forehead from one side to the other; as your hand is nearly finished, lay the other hand on the forehead and stroke in the opposite direction. Repeat several times and imagine you are stroking tension and worry away from your partner.

6

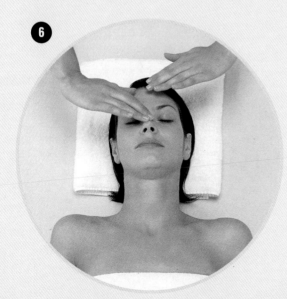

7

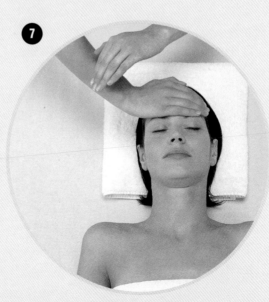

⑧ Steadying your fingertips on the sides of the head, place your thumbs on the centre of the forehead, just above the eyebrows. Lean slightly into your thumbs, and hold this pressure for a few seconds. Release, move your thumbs further apart, still above the eyebrows, and lean in again. Move the thumbs along, leaning into them several times, just above eyebrow level. Then bring your thumbs back to the centre, halfway up the forehead, and work another row across the forehead; then work a third row just under the hairline. ⑨ With fingers on the sides of the head, bring together the muscles at the base of your two

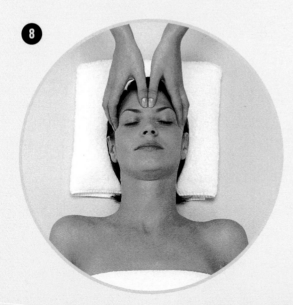

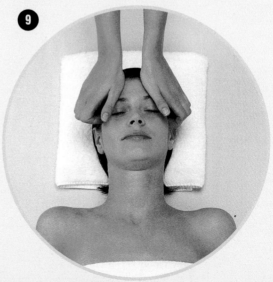

thumbs, resting in the middle of the forehead. Smooth your thumb muscles apart, out to the temples. Now extend your fingers to cradle your partner's chin, then draw your fingers back up the sides of the face, and repeat the whole movement several times. It's worth persevering with this beautiful move: when you get the hang of it, it is a profoundly peaceful motion, almost like rocking. ⑩ With fingers apart, press firmly into your partner's scalp and draw small circles. Try to move the scalp itself, not the hair. ⑪ Finish with a simple hold: one hand on your partner's upper chest and the other on their crown.

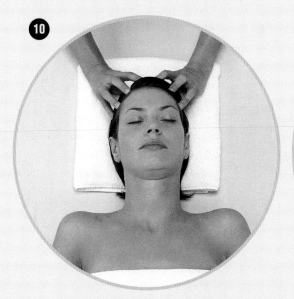

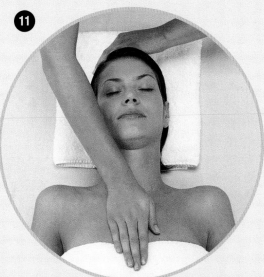

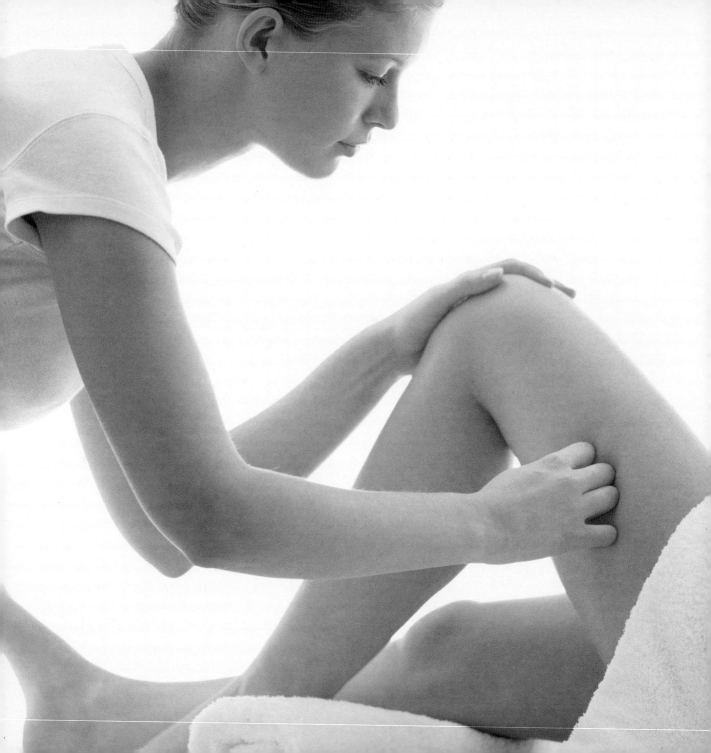

CHAPTER 4:
Easy Variations

The techniques and routines that you have learned so far have equipped you to give good, simple massages that are suitable for most people. In this chapter I will show you how to adapt and expand your massage skills for special situations. For example, if you are massaging a pregnant woman, an elderly person or someone who is training for a marathon, their needs will be very different.

You can assess the needs of your massage partner from different perspectives. First of all you need to address the physical practicality of determining the kind of massage that will suit them, bearing in mind their particular state of health. Second, you need to make an empathic appraisal of the person; think about who they are, and how they may feel, perhaps living in an old body, or being pregnant, or convalescing. Be assured that as you practise your massage skills and develop your awareness of their special needs, you will gradually build confidence in giving a treatment tailor-made just for them.

Massaging pregnant women

Pregnancy is an extraordinary time in a woman's life. Her body is changing, week by week, providing a complex life-support system for a tiny being. Broadly speaking, pregnancy falls into three main phases, or trimesters, each of which lasts around three months. Massage can be a wonderfully supportive and therapeutic treatment to receive throughout pregnancy. However, it is vital that you work safely when massaging someone who is pregnant. Check that the expectant mother has consulted her midwife about receiving massage, and work gently, using only smooth, flowing movements.

During the first trimester the expectant mother's body feels much less predictable than before – maybe queasy or maybe not, sometimes exhausted and sometimes fine – aware that this is the time where a pregnancy may not yet be stable. The second trimester is usually a time of well-being – the pregnant woman has plenty of energy for normal life, glowing skin and increased confidence in the pregnancy. The third trimester is when she begins to feel physically unwieldy as the baby grows quite sizeable. This stage puts the most strain on the mother's body. She might suffer backache, as her spine is pulled forward by the weight of the baby, or swollen ankles as her circulation is affected, or sometimes dry skin.

During the first trimester you should apply massage very gently. Avoid the abdominal area, and massage the lower back only with the lightest of touches. Do not use essential oils during this stage.

During the second and third trimesters, as the baby grows, the mother-to-be will find it increasingly difficult to lie on her front. Also, it is best if she doesn't lie flat on her back as this can become uncomfortable after a short while. It is possible to massage her lying on her side, but it is much easier to massage her while she is sitting. While she may not be able to receive a full-body massage, she can still have massage on many different parts of the body (the face, back and shoulders, hands, arms, legs and feet) and feel soothed, relaxed and revitalized by it.

The secret ingredient for massage during this time is numerous pillows. For a back massage the woman can sit on a stool or chair in front of a table that has three pillows in a pile on top of it. Ask her to lean her head and arms onto the pillows, and be sure to take your time over her comfort. For massage elsewhere on her body, she can sit in a chair or on a massage table or a futon – as long as she is not lying absolutely flat. Prop her up with plenty of pillows for comfort.

Some essential oils can be safely used in the second and third trimester, but some are contraindicated. Always check with a qualified aromatherapist if you wish to give a massage with essential oils to someone who is pregnant.

Massaging babies

When a baby is born they leave a place of total safety and warmth, where every need has been answered and their body has been cradled constantly. It's almost impossible to imagine how huge the change must feel once they enter the world, even when the birth has been straightforward. If the birth has been difficult, their cortisol levels (stress hormones) can be a hundred times higher than those of an adult man having a heart attack.

Touch is more effective than anything else at relieving stress in a newborn. Cradling and breast-feeding a baby immediately after birth is greatly calming, and employing massage from the first hours is a truly loving and effective way of helping a baby to relax.

When you give a baby a massage the room needs to be very warm, as they should be naked. Sit on the floor, with your back supported, and your legs straight out in front of you. Place a thick towel on your legs and lay your baby on top, their feet toward you. Use a good-quality sunflower oil or olive oil. As you begin, don't worry if your baby cries at first – they will soon settle into deep enjoyment. Please note: do not massage a baby if they have a full stomach.

The massage techniques you use are not nearly as important as paying attention to really focusing your whole self on your baby: speak with your eyes, your smile, and through your hands, and let the whole experience flow from your heart. See how your hands can adapt to their tiny body. You may feel clumsy at first, but keep going. Use slow, gentle strokes: you will find moves that seem to fit.

However, if you would like to follow a loose baby-massage routine, you can try the following moves. Begin by laying the fingers of both of your hands on their little chest, then smooth them sideways, as though you were smoothing open a book; draw your fingers down the sides of their ribcage and back to the centre. Then, with alternate hands, smooth your hand from their hip diagonally across their body to their opposite shoulder; and as you reach the shoulder, begin with your other hand from the opposite hip. Glide your fingers over one shoulder and lightly clasp your fingers round their arm. Gently "milk" their arm upward toward their hand. Follow with your other hand and repeat several times. Then, supporting your baby's wrist, use your thumbs to massage their palms. Massage each finger. "Milk" the little legs as you did the arms, with alternate hands; massage the tiny ankles and use your thumbs for the soles of their feet.

Then lay them sideways across your legs and turn them on their tummy. Cup their buttocks with one hand and stroke their back, peacefully, slowly, time after time. Relax into giving everything to this tiny being. Trust yourself to learn how they need to be touched.

Massaging the elderly

Massage has many particular benefits for elderly people. Regular treatments can alleviate minor ills, such as aches and pains, and can support the mobility of joints, improve circulation, relax chronic tension and improve the immune system.

Remember that many old people have lived with a family, but are now alone. Maybe touch was an easy, natural part of life for decades, but partners have died and children moved away. The caring touch and physical communication experienced during massage can be a real boost to them, especially if they are suffering from loneliness. Sometimes you may be the only person who touches them with intimacy and tenderness. It is always a

privilege to give a massage; when the body you are treating is old, massage it with respect for the lifetime that has been lived in it.

Before you start massaging, as always, make sure that none of the contraindications apply. If in doubt about any aspect of their health in relation to massage, ask them to check with their doctor that it is suitable for them to receive a treatment. If the person you wish to massage is thin, keep the massage room extra warm, and have plenty of towels and a light blanket to hand: thin people of all ages easily get cold during massage.

Some older people may be comfortable with the idea of a full-body massage and the undressing that this requires. However, many older people will not, and this is why massage for the elderly often focuses on areas such as the hands and feet, neck and shoulders, or face. This will still be highly beneficial. If, however, they would like a full-body massage, take extra care to protect their privacy while they are changing, and be ready to help them onto the couch or floor. They may be less mobile than they once were, and joints may be arthritic. Have pillows to hand to support their knees or head; take time over comfort.

If they would prefer to receive a back massage only, seat them on a stool, facing a table with three pillows piled up. Have them lean forward, resting their head and arms on the pillows. Make sure they are comfortable.

Older skin is thinner, drier and more fragile, so you will need to choose a rich, emollient massage oil that will nourish the skin (see chapter 6, Easy Massage Oils). The addition of appropriate essential oils (see pp.138–139) will add to the pleasure of the massage, but stick to a dilution of 1% (1 drop of essential oil to 5ml carrier oil, see pp.127–129). Usually, for an old person, stroking will be the best technique to use, with a little gentle kneading where appropriate. Keep checking that the pressure feels right to them. Remember to apply only featherlight stroking over varicose veins. At the end of the treatment, help them up without rushing, and offer them a glass of water or a cup of tea.

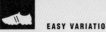

Massage after exercise

A muscle does two things: it contracts and it relaxes. The physical action of moving our bones is achieved by the contraction of skeletal muscle. These muscles work in pairs: one, called the agonist, contracts to create a movement, while the other, the antagonist, stretches to accommodate the movement. To check or stop the movement, the antagonist in turn contracts, and this pulls the agonist back to a relaxed state. Thus, the two muscles work in a reciprocal, complementary way, and this relationship is coordinated in the brain. Imagine how many pairs of muscles must be working, without you being conscious of it, for you to dance, run, perform in sports, or even just be able to walk.

Following extended physical exertion, the muscles are likely to be laden with the metabolic byproducts of muscle use. Muscles need glucose and oxygen to give them the energy to contract. For example, when you start running, the body responds to this muscle activity by increasing the heart and breathing rates, and by releasing glucose into the bloodstream. As the muscle works, waste products are produced. Continuous muscle contraction keeps squeezing the blood and lymph vessels within the muscle, pumping the cleansing fluids through, increasing the flow back to the heart or lymph nodes.

Intensive exercise can mean that metabolic waste builds up within the muscle; it may not have been possible for the excretion process to keep pace. Cooling down properly will help: stretching the body keeps the blood and lymph moving through the muscles, continuing the clean-up process. Massage is an additional effective way of helping the body shift waste matter from the muscles.

Ideally, give the massage soon after the exercise session, or at least the same day. Your aim is to encourage the circulation of blood and lymph.

Say you are massaging someone training for a marathon; you will probably be working mainly on the legs and buttocks. After the training session, start by warming the area with stroking, then begin kneading; this mobilizes the tissues and begins to increase the circulation. You can carry on kneading for some time; you will feel the tissues become more pliable. If the muscles are not too tender, move on to knuckling fairly deeply, checking the pressure feels right for your partner. Then begin running your knuckles in firm lines, following the grain of the muscle (see diagram, p.19), working in the overall direction of the heart. You will be helping to pump blood and lymph through the muscle, and so removing waste.

Caution: Occasionally, muscle tightness may be protecting a weakness or an injury. If you or your partner think this could be the case, refer them to someone trained to deal with sports injuries.

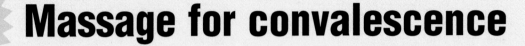

Massage for convalescence

Massage can often be a real boost to a person during a period of convalescence as it can help the body to cultivate the optimum conditions for its own healing. Relaxing, soothing strokes can ease tension and gently boost the circulation.

Generally, however, you should not massage someone who is battling an infection, because their body is fighting illness and they probably won't feel like receiving a massage. Also, those giving massage should not risk infection. The exception is if they have a long-term infection that cannot be passed on during massage. For example, it is usually fine to massage someone with HIV/AIDS – indeed treatment can boost the immune system in such cases.

When someone is recovering from a serious illness, always ask the opinion and advice of their doctor before giving them massage, to make sure that it will be beneficial. If someone is very frail, it is usually possible to give them a hand or foot massage if nothing else, and this alone can help boost the healing process. If a person has to spend weeks in bed owing to illness, and there is a risk of pressure sores, massage can be a vital prophylactic. Seek medical advice concerning where, how often and how best to massage to keep the patient's skin intact. A bed-ridden person may also suffer from stiff joints and muscle wastage; massage can support joint mobility and help to maintain good circulation in the extremities.

If you are massaging someone who has recently had surgery, it's important that you don't attempt to massage new scar tissue. In the first weeks after an operation, you can give massage elsewhere on the body but only very gently, monitoring how the patient feels afterward. It can help greatly with their sleep and relaxation, which in turn can aid recovery.

If someone has a broken bone set in plaster, massaging the parts of a limb that are not plastered can help the circulation in the whole area. When the plaster is removed, there is always some muscle wastage; and people are sometimes horrified by the way dry skin has built up and comes away in flakes. Careful washing and drying of the area will remove some of the dead skin cells, then gentle massage will help the circulation and also begin to restore skin condition. Ideally this should be repeated daily for two weeks.

Using essential oils in your massage blend can be an extra help during convalescence, but if the person is elderly, fragile or taking medication, stick to a dilution of 1% (1 drop of oil to 5ml of carrier oil), and seek the advice of an aromatherapist on your choice of oils.

Finally, massage can provide an exquisite quality of care for a person who is dying. Gentle massage of the hands or feet can be relaxing and soothing, and can feel as though you have the privilege of anointing the dying person before the next part of their journey.

Massaging delicate skin

We often forget that our skin is an organ of the body. In fact it is the largest organ we have, and vital to our well-being. It has several key functions. First, as it is largely impermeable, the skin keeps out water, bacteria and other micro-organisms. Second, it is part of our heat-regulation system: when we're hot, we release sweat through our skin's pores in order to cool down; and when we're cold, tiny hairs on our skin stand on end to conserve our body heat. Sweating is also part of our waste-disposal system – waste leaves the body not only via the excretory organs but also via the skin (and the breath). Finally, the skin is covered in nerve endings that tell us about our environment, relaying heat, cold, touch, pressure and pain.

Skin is usually self-lubricating and self-repairing, and elastic and mobile. Dry skin is less good at self-lubricating, and therefore thinner and less elastic. Sensitive skin reacts over-easily to external irritants, such as washing powder, cosmetics and some fabrics, resulting in it becoming red and itchy. This can be exacerbated by internal factors such as stress, which can be a trigger for eczema.

When massaging dry skin avoid techniques that use excessive stretching or friction. Stroking and kneading are fine but apply them more gently than usual. Use a rich, emollient oil, which will lubricate the skin and leave it soothed and supple. When massaging sensitive skin it is best to use plain, good-quality vegetable oils: these are least likely to cause irritation. Chapter 6, Easy Massage Oils, suggests oils that are particularly helpful for sensitive skin. You should use essential oils only with great care on sensitive skin, and in a 1% dilution (1 drop to 5ml carrier oil). Some essential oils can irritate sensitive skin, so consult an aromatherapist about the choice of oils before you use any.

With problem skin of other kinds, it may still be fine to give massage depending on the exact nature of the skin condition. If the person concerned has the highly infectious condition impetigo, you should not massage them at all, to avoid any risk of cross-infection. Some other skin conditions are infectious, but to a lesser degree, and you can usually massage elsewhere on the body if you wish. These include cold sores, warts, verrucae, ringworm, athlete's foot and scabies. However, remember to wash your hands and towels thoroughly afterward.

If the person is suffering a non-infectious skin condition, such as eczema, dermatitis, psoriasis, acne rosacea or vitiligo, it's fine to massage, but be aware that they may feel sensitive about their appearance. Be matter-of-fact the first time you massage them, and say that you would like to keep checking that the massage feels comfortable. Explain that you will use an oil that is helpful to sensitive skin. If the skin is very disturbed (but unbroken), simply use gentle stroking and nothing else.

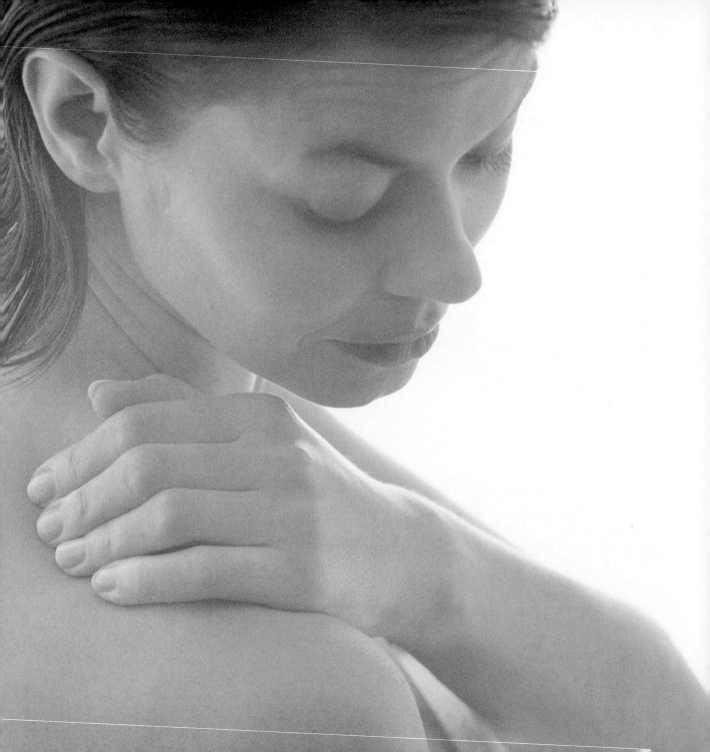

CHAPTER 5:
Easy Self-massage

Gathering the skills associated with massage is a deeply pleasurable process, both for you and your massage recipients. As you become skilful at using different techniques, and at promoting relaxation and health in your massage partners, there is a bonus waiting: you can also use your skills for self-massage to support your own well-being. And, as we have already discussed, caring for yourself is a key requirement for anyone who gives massage to others.

This chapter shows you how to give yourself a range of short, effective self-massages. Some you can use to keep yourself well: for example, if you know you are prone to stress headaches, try the treatment on pages 104–105 as a preventative. Others will help you to alleviate the symptoms of a range of common ailments.

Headaches

Headaches are often caused by chronic tension in the neck, the jaw and around the eyes. When we are under pressure, we often tighten the musculature in these areas without even realizing we are doing it. Taking a few minutes to release this tension can make a big difference in the prevention and relief of headaches.

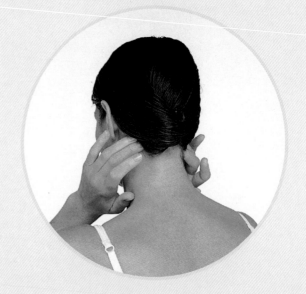

TIP: When you are feeling under pressure, it is well worth taking a few minutes to give yourself this routine before you get a headache – if necessary do it several times in a day. If you are really committed about doing this, it is very likely the headache will never arrive.

1 Inhale slowly and deeply and, as you release the breath, consciously soften your tight jaw. Take your fingertips behind your ears and find the edge of your skull. Press just under the bone, working in tiny circles. Work your way along the base of your skull until your fingers meet. If you find places that feel tender, remain circling on them for a little while longer. Keep your jaw soft.

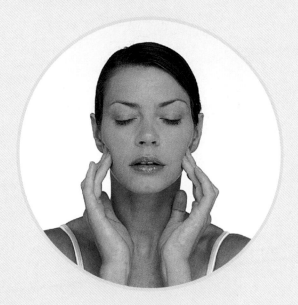

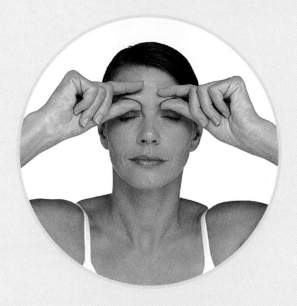

2 Take your fingertips to the hinges of your jaw. Press in firmly, moving your fingertips in tiny circles. As you do this, allow your breath to deepen, with a good, releasing outbreath. You may find that you yawn involuntarily. Work all around the hinges of your jaw, pressing as deeply as is comfortable.

3 Place your thumbs just under the inner corners of your eyebrows, and drop your head forward slightly so that your thumbs are supporting it. Keep your jaw soft and continue to breathe slowly and deeply. Now pinch your way along your eyebrows, using thumbs and forefingers. Finally place your fingertips on your temples and gently work in circles, with your eyes closed.

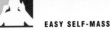
Sinus problems

If you suffer from blocked sinuses, you will know exactly how debilitating it can be. Massage, especially using an appropriate essential oil blend (see p.138), can help to keep your sinuses clear. Give yourself this treatment frequently if you have a head cold or hayfever.

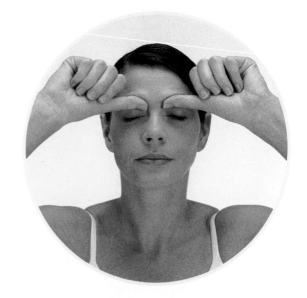

TIP: If you are using the Decongestant essential oil blend (see p.138), smooth a little of the blend under your nose when you begin this treatment so that you are inhaling the oils while you give yourself the massage.

1 Spread a teaspoonful of the Decongestant essential oil blend, or your usual massage oil, above your eyebrows, across your cheekbones and down the sides of your nose. Be very careful not to get oil in your eyes. Start by massaging with your thumbs under the inner ends of your eyebrows, pressing as firmly as is comfortable.

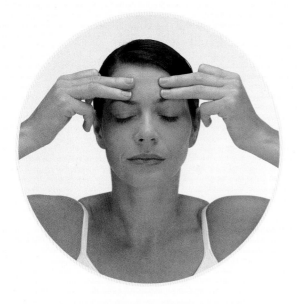

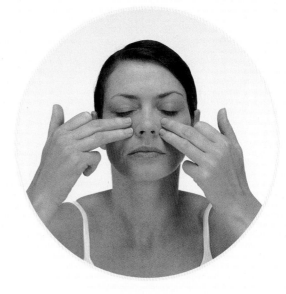

2 Now with the tips of your tallest fingers and ring fingers, massage your forehead above the inner ends of your eyebrows on both sides. Press with small, firm circles, working around the sinus area. To finish massaging this area, use the fingertips of both hands to stroke outward across your forehead, away from the centre.

3 With your tallest fingers and ring fingers, press down either side of your nose, starting about a finger's width down from the edge of your eye socket. Press with small, firm circles, as firmly as is comfortable, part way across your cheeks, following the contour of the eye socket. Finish with a couple of gentle strokes outward across your cheeks.

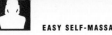

Eyestrain

Anyone who works at a computer, or who performs other tasks that require constant close focusing, is likely to have tired eyes at the end of the day. This short massage takes only a few minutes, and is extremely helpful for relaxing the area around the eyes. Try doing it several times a day, to help you to avoid eyestrain.

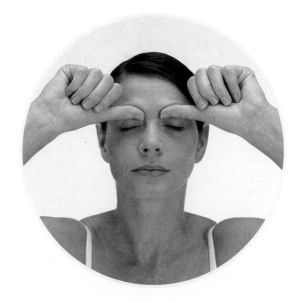

TIP: When you are doing close work, look away regularly and focus on something in the distance. Also, if you can do it without alarming others, raise your eyebrows and open your eyes wide, then relax and smile. These simple exercises all help to relax the tiny muscles around the eyes.

1 Put your elbows on a table and place your thumbs under the inner ends of your eyebrows. Close your eyes, and relax your neck so that your thumbs take the weight of your head. Make tiny circles on the spot with your thumbs. Breathe in, then release the breath right out. Now pinch along your eyebrows with your thumbs and forefingers.

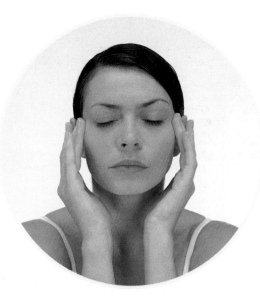

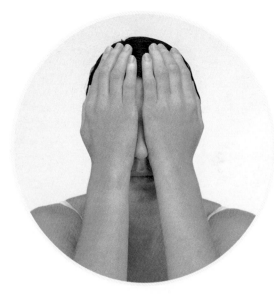

2 With eyes still closed, take your fingertips just below your temples, on the same level as your eyes. Press firmly, and as you do this relax your jaw, breathe in again then release the breath right out. Begin to draw small, firm circles with your fingertips in this position. Keep your breathing deep and relaxed.

3 To end place your palms over your eyes, with your elbows still on the table. Let the weight of your head be held by your palms. Fit the palms so well over your eyes that you see nothing but black. This relaxes the eyes. Hold this position for a minute or so, keeping your jaw soft and your breathing relaxed.

Tense shoulders

We all hold tension in our shoulders, and it happens insidiously. Right now, take a breath, and with your outbreath see if your shoulders fall a little. You'll probably find they do. This massage helps loosen tight shoulders during a difficult day.

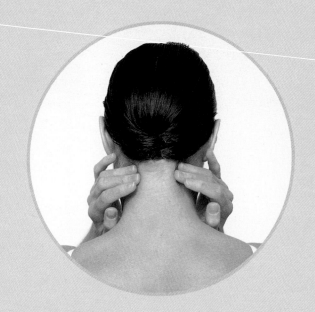

TIP: The tension in your shoulders is linked to your neck, which in turn is linked to your jaw. To ease this tension throughout the day it helps regularly to take a breath in, consciously soften your jaw and slowly breathe right out, dropping your shoulders down as you go.

1 Sit comfortably in a chair that supports your back. Place your fingertips on both sides of the vertebrae at the back of your head, and press in, making small, firm circles. Move the circles out along the bottom edge of your skull. You may find this easier if you drop your head back a little.

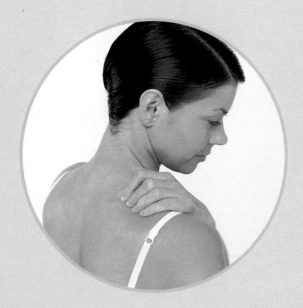

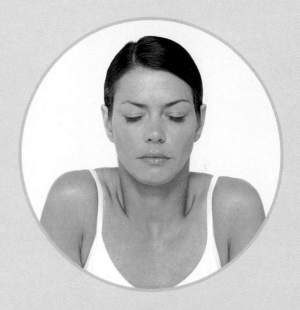

2 With your left hand, locate the muscle on top of your right shoulder. With your palm on the front of your shoulder and your fingers on the back, squeeze and lift the muscle several times. Then use your fingertips to circle deeply into the muscle. Circle longer on any particularly tight areas that you find. Repeat, using your right hand on your left shoulder.

3 Now imagine that you have chalk on the outside of each shoulder, and slowly draw four large circles forward and four circles backward with both shoulders at the same time. Finally draw your shoulders up as high as you can, then very slowly let them fall until they have dropped right down and are fully relaxed. The slower you do this the better.

Nervous stomach

Many people suffer from a nervous stomach when under pressure. Whether this manifests as cramps, diarrhoea, constipation or wind, this treatment can help, particularly if you use a calming and warming essential oil blend (see p.139).

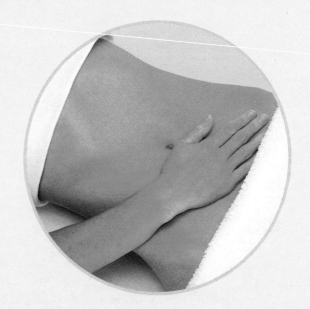

TIP: Give yourself this treatment when you're not in a rush. Rushing tends to make nervous stomachs worse. Organize your schedule so that the important things in your life can happen without panic. Remember that, in the great scheme of things, daily upsets often aren't that bad.

1 Lying flat, spread massage oil over your abdomen. Using a relaxed palm and fingers, begin to massage in a slow, large circle clockwise round your stomach. Close your eyes and soften your jaw. Keep the rhythm peaceful and try to slow and deepen your breathing. Send the message through your hands: calm.

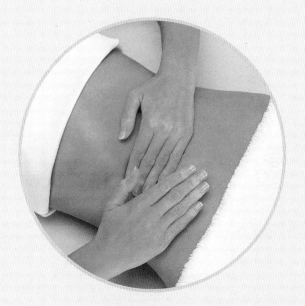

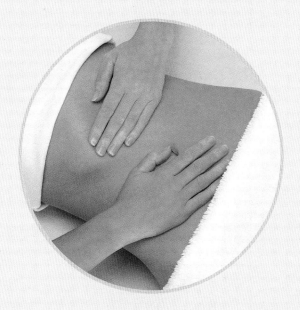

2 Using your hands alternately, stroke up the right side of your abdomen several times. Now with alternate hands, stroke across the top of your abdomen several times, and then down the left side of your abdomen the same way. This follows the direction of your colon. Keep thinking all the while: calm.

3 Now move back to slow circling again; and this time, work with both your hands. Your main hand does slow, big, clockwise circles as before, and your other hand follows. When your second hand encounters the first, just slide it over the top of your first hand, and keep both hands circling. Use slow movements and keep thinking: calm. Do this slow, relaxed circling for several minutes. Finish with a long, slow outbreath.

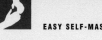

Constipation

This is an effective treatment for ordinary constipation. The pressures of everyday life can often result in constipation, because of tension, or a rushed diet, or missed meals. This treatment is best performed in the evening. Note: if you suffer from bowel disease, liaise with your doctor before giving yourself this massage.

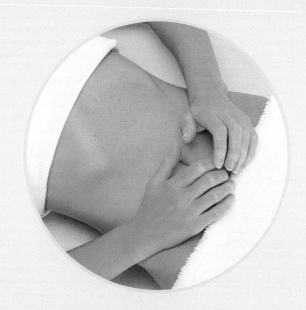

TIP: It's difficult to get constipated if you drink enough water. Aim for two litres (three and a half pints) a day, apart from other drinks. Eat regularly and remember to consume at least five portions of fruit or vegetables daily to help maintain optimum bowel health.

1 Lying flat, spread oil over your abdomen. Begin by massaging over your ascending and descending colon (see p.21): place your hands flat so that your fingertips nearly meet at your navel, then press into the sides of your stomach with the heels of your hands, and use your hands to massage the area in small, deep circles, working as firmly as is comfortable up the sides of the front of your abdomen.

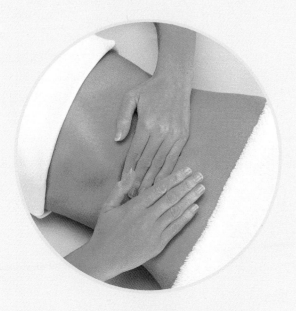

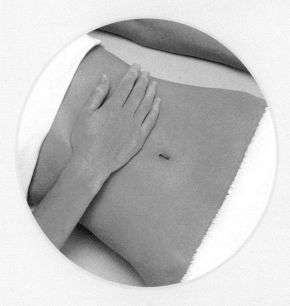

2 Using the flats of your fingers, working with alternate hands, massage firmly up your right side (the ascending colon), across your upper midriff (transverse colon) and down your left side (descending colon). Take your time, pressing as firmly as is comfortable, and keep your stomach muscles relaxed. Always work your fingers in a clockwise direction.

3 Place the palm of one hand on your stomach, with relaxed fingers, and begin to circle clockwise. Press as firmly as is comfortable with your stomach muscles relaxed, and keep the pressure constant, circling clockwise in the space bounded by your ribs and hip bones. Use the heel and palm of your hand and be firm. Finish by relaxing your hand below the navel.

Period pains

This simple massage can really help with aching cramps, particularly if you use an appropriate oil blend with warming, calming essential oils (see p.139). If you have time have a warm bath before this treatment, as warmth will begin to relax the uterine muscle that is cramping and causing the pain.

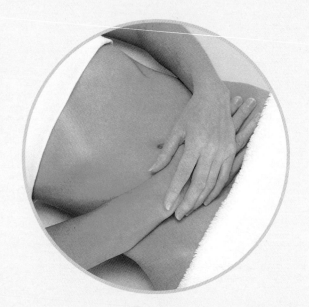

TIP: If possible, after you have given yourself this treatment, lie down with a warm wheatbag on your lower tummy. The warmth is comforting and will also help your skin to continue absorbing the oils.

1 Lying on your back, oil your hands and, to begin, simply lay your hands, one on top of the other, on your lower tummy just above the pubic bone. Keep your breathing calm and even, and wait for the warmth of your hands to begin sinking into the cramping area.

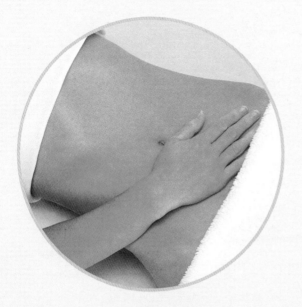

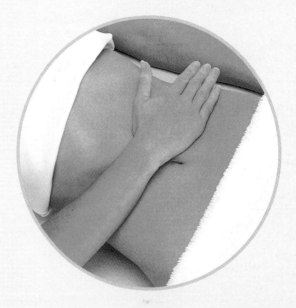

2 Very gently, begin to make small circles with one relaxed palm, keeping the circle below your navel. Don't use any pressure, keep your breathing calm and remind yourself that the cramps will pass soon. Continue this palm circling for at least five to ten minutes. The warmth of your hand encourages your skin to absorb the oils.

3 As the cramps begin to ease, gradually make the circles bigger, stroking clockwise round your abdomen with your palm and relaxed fingers. Keep the movement very slow and peaceful, with no pressure, as you relax the whole area. Finish by laying your hands back above the pubic bone for a few moments.

Nervous exhaustion

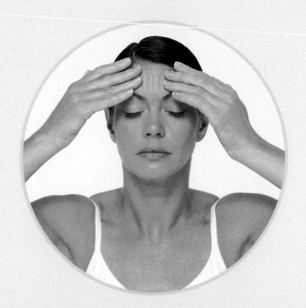

You should take this kind of exhaustion seriously – it undermines your immune system, quite apart from destroying your pleasure in life. This massage will help you to unwind, so that you can rest and take stock of life.

TIP: If you find yourself emotionally and physically exhausted, it's time to stop and take a look at your life. Your health is precious, and exhaustion undermines it. Examine your life–work balance, and consider where you need to make changes; and learn to guard your relaxation time like a Rottweiler.

1 First, close your eyes, breathe out, breathe right in, then expel a long, releasing breath. Using a calming oil blend (see p.139), gently oil your face, the back of your neck and the tops of your shoulders. With your fingertips, massage small circles over your forehead and temples. Consciously soften your jaw and keep your breathing relaxed.

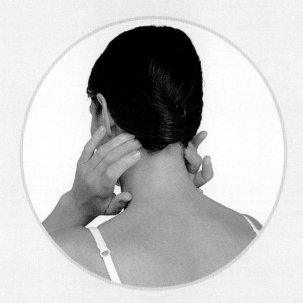

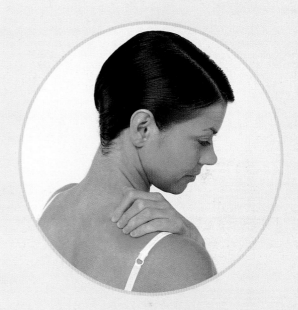

2 Massage the back of your neck with your fingertips; make tiny circles under the edge of your skull, working from behind the ears to the top of your spine. Keep your eyes closed and your jaw soft. Work your fingers over the back of your neck. Remind yourself that life will not always be this frantic.

3 Take your right hand to your left shoulder, with your palm on the front, and your fingers on the back. Squeeze the tense muscles here until you feel them soften. Repeat on the other side. Now lay your palm on your upper chest, and, moving in slow circles, send yourself the message: I deserve to relax. Do this for two or three minutes, keeping your jaw soft. Finish with a long outbreath.

Aching feet

Our feet are a miracle of engineering, and one that we tend to take for granted. If you have been rushing around all day, this massage will help to restore your aching feet. If you have time first soap your feet, soak them in warm water for five minutes, then dry them.

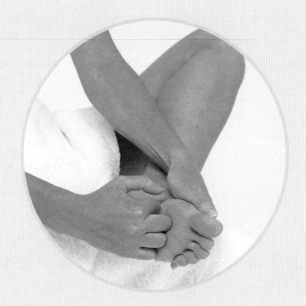

TIP: When you have given your feet this massage, put them up for a while, to get the full benefit of the treatment. If they are swollen, lie with your feet higher than your body for ten minutes.

1 Lay your left foot on a towel on your right knee. Oil your foot and ankle with a cooling oil blend (see p.138). Lay your left hand on top of your foot to brace it, and with your right hand, knuckle the sole of your foot all over, working quite deeply.

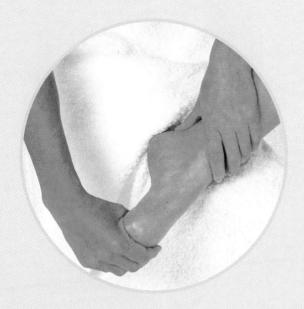

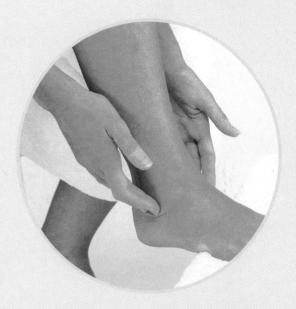

2 Hold your foot with one hand and firmly massage each of your toes with the other hand. Next, hold all your toes in your hand and bend them down a little as though pointing them. Then take your toes between your hands and fan them out, opening the space between each one.

3 Now hold your heel in one hand and stroke the top of your foot firmly from toes to ankle several times. Massage firmly round your ankle bones with the fingertips of both hands. Finally wrap both hands around your ankle and squeeze it upward several times, before stroking up toward your calf. Repeat these moves on your other foot. End by putting your feet up, literally, for a few minutes if you can.

Insomnia

When the brain gets too busy or anxiety levels are high, sleep can be elusive. If this is happening to you, organize yourself for the next day, then make your evening peaceful, even boring. Have a warm (not hot) bath and, just before bedtime, give yourself this simple massage, using a calming and unwinding oil blend (see p.139).

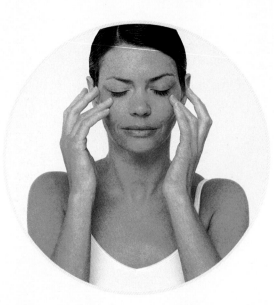

TIP: Add 6 or 8 drops of lavender essential oil to your bath to begin the unwinding process; then at bedtime sprinkle a few drops of lavender oil on a tissue and lay it beside your pillow. Lavender has been shown to promote more relaxed sleep.

1 First stroke the tension from around your eyes. Close your eyes and use your fingertips to make tiny circles all around the edge of your eye sockets. (Take care not to get oil in your eyes.) Move the tiny circles out to your temples. Keep your jaw soft and let your breathing be slow and calm.

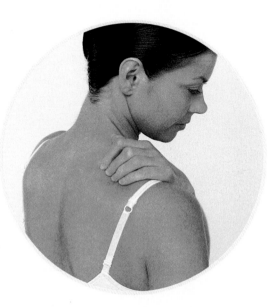

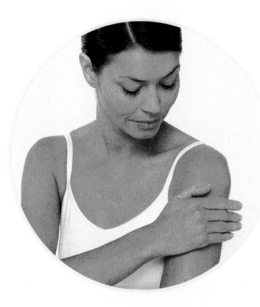

2 Now squeeze the tension away from your shoulders. Take the top of one shoulder in your opposite hand, palm on the front and fingers on the back; lift and squeeze the muscle, starting by the base of your neck and moving out across your shoulder. Keep your jaw soft and your breathing calm. Repeat on the other side.

3 Now stroke the last of the tension away. Lay your right hand on the left side of your neck. Smooth your hand down your neck, along your left shoulder, down your whole arm and off at your fingertips. Do this several times, imagining you are sweeping away tension. Repeat on the other side. Keep your jaw soft and your face totally relaxed as you go to bed.

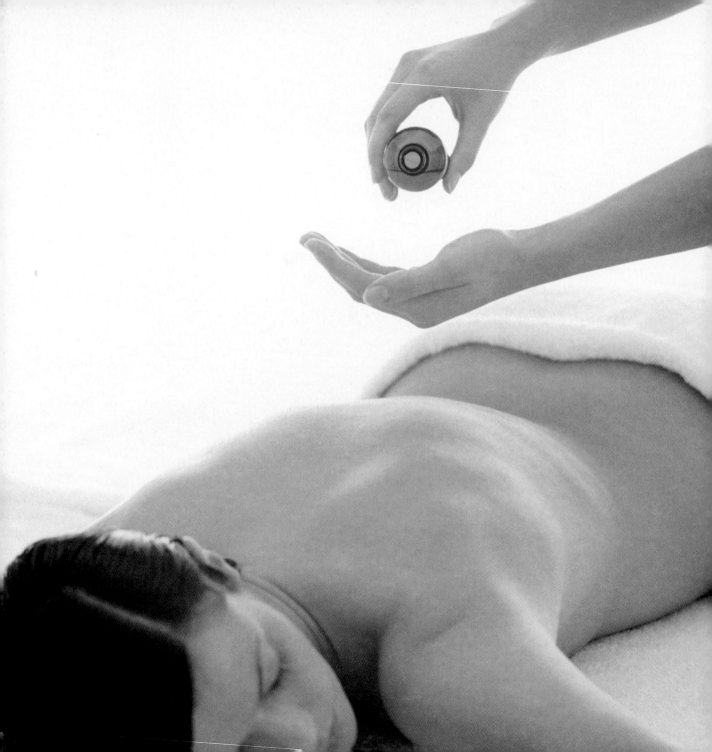

CHAPTER 6:
Easy Massage Oils

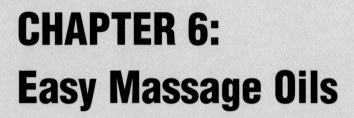

When you pour oil into your palm, ready to massage another person, you are continuing an ancient healing tradition. Centuries ago healers would have taken oil pressed from olives, almonds or other plants, spread it on their hands and begun to massage, exactly as you are doing. There is a vast array of plant oils that can be used for massage, all obtained from the bounty of nature.

In this chapter I will introduce you to some of the best carrier oils available – both good basic oils for everyday use and special oils that are ideal for particular conditions – and offer guidelines for buying and storing them. I will also direct your first steps in the blending of essential oils into your massage mix; you will find clear advice on safety, and a range of effective, safe and aromatic massage blend "recipes" for you to try for yourself.

Using massage oils

The oil, or oils, that you use for a massage are a basic part of the treatment you give, but they are also a part that offers you the chance to tailor your treatment to the individual recipient, thereby enhancing even further the healing experience of the massage. Where you buy and store your oils, how you blend them, and how you use them safely are all crucial factors that can help you to give your massage partner the best possible treatment.

BUYING OILS

The quality of an oil depends in the first instance on the quality of the original plant. Factors such as the soil and climate in which it was grown, and whether the plant was sprayed with pesticides, wild or cultivated, all affect its standard, as do aspects of its journey from plant to bottle. Here it is helpful to know how the oil was extracted from the plant, whether chemicals were added, and how it was shipped and stored. All of these things can affect the quality of the oil you buy, so I advise that you make every effort to purchase your oils from a knowledgeable supplier who is committed to high quality, and who can tell you something about the oils that they sell.

STORING OILS

All oils, whether carrier oils or essential oils, must be stored in dark glass bottles, tightly capped, and kept in a cool, dark place. A refrigerator is ideal. This is because UV light and heat greatly speeds up their degradation, and exposure to light and heat will shorten an oil's shelf life. Most oils have a shelf life of two years if kept in the refrigerator, and half this time if kept in non-refrigerated but cool and dark conditions.

Keep essential oils out of the reach of children as they are highly concentrated substances that may be harmful if they are ingested or applied neat to the skin. They are also flammable, so should always be kept away from naked flames. Finally, take care not to place essential oils on polished or painted surfaces – any spilled drops will leave a stain – and always wipe up a spill immediately.

BLENDING OILS

Adding essential oils to a carrier oil creates a beautiful aromatic mix that can bring another dimension to massage. However, before including essential oils in your massage mix, it's vital that you prepare them to the correct dilution and find out if any oils may be contraindicated for the person receiving treatment. If you are unsure about any aspect of using essential oils on your massage partner, seek the advice of a qualified aromatherapist.

To make an essential oil blend you will need a small, clean plastic measuring pot, and a stirring spoon. First measure out your chosen carrier oil. (For more details on possible

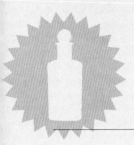

carrier oils see pages 130–137.) As a rough guide to the amount of oil you will need, for a back massage use 2tsp (10ml), and for a full-body massage use between 4tsp (20ml) and 6tsp (30ml), depending on the size of the person you wish to massage. Next you will need to add the correct number of drops of essential oil. The standard dilution is 2%. This means that for each 1tsp (5ml) of carrier oil, you should add a total of 2 drops of essential oil. There are certain situations where a weaker dilution is appropriate – see the Safety Guidelines below. Remember that it will not only be your massage partner who benefits from the aromatic effects of using essential oils as part of a massage – as the giver of the massage you, too, will enjoy the aromas and effects of such a treatment. See pages 138–139 for some essential oil blends for you to try.

SAFETY GUIDELINES FOR BLENDING

• A standard 2% dilution is suitable for anyone in good health over the age of 12. For children aged between three and 12 years, you should use a dilution of 1% if treating them with a massage blend containing essential oils. Infants between the ages of six months and three years can be massaged with blends containing tiny amounts of essential oils, but I would advise that blends for this age group be prepared by a qualified aromatherapist for you to use at home. Babies under the age of six months should be massaged with a carrier oil alone – use a good-quality sunflower or olive oil for this, and avoid oils that are nut-based.

• If your massage partner is pregnant, it's safest to avoid using essential oils during the first trimester altogether. Thereafter, consult an aromatherapist, as some essential oils should be avoided throughout pregnancy. Dilution of essential oil blends for pregnant women should be 1% or less. This means that you need to add only one drop of essential oil for every 1tsp (5ml) of carrier oil being used.

• You should use a dilution of 1% for essential oil blends that you wish to use on anyone who is elderly, frail, or who has dry or sensitive skin. All of these groups of people can show greater skin sensitivity to some of the properties of the oils.

• If you use any citrus oils in an essential oil blend, advise the person receiving the massage that these increase skin sensitivity to the sun, so they should take care to avoid the sun and sunbeds on the day of treatment.

• If your partner is using homeopathy, consult a homeopath before using essential oils in the massage treatment. Some oils are thought to antidote homeopathic remedies.

• If your massage partner has epilepsy or high blood pressure, consult their doctor and an aromatherapist before using essential oils on them, as you need to avoid using those oils that have stimulating properties.

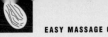

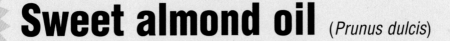

Sweet almond oil (*Prunus dulcis*)

Native to the Middle East, the almond has been cultivated for thousands of years. It is now also grown in the Mediterranean and California. Around 5m (15ft) tall, it has pink or white blossom in spring. The fruits contain almond kernels and resemble small, green apricots.

Sweet almond oil is one of the most popular vegetable oils for massage. It is pale yellow in colour, slightly viscous and very oily, and has a faint sweet smell. The best-quality oil is obtained by cold-pressing the kernels.

THERAPEUTIC PROPERTIES

If you buy only one oil for massage, choose sweet almond. It is easy to use and suitable for all skin types. An excellent emollient, it alleviates and nourishes dry skin. It helps to soothe inflammation, and can temporarily relieve itching caused by eczema, psoriasis, dermatitis and dry skin conditions. It is also a good oil to use as a base to blend with other oils: it is moderately priced, and fairly neutral in viscosity and aroma.

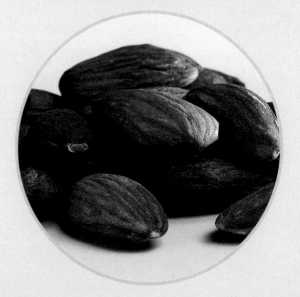

Jojoba oil (*Symmondsia sinensis*)

Jojoba is a small shrub with leathery, blue-green leaves, that grows up to 2m (7ft) in height. It can be found in the desert regions of Southern California, Arizona and northwest Mexico. The hulls of the jojoba's fruit turn from green to brown, then crack and allow the seed to fall to the ground. Jojoba seeds look like coffee beans.

Jojoba is not actually an oil but a golden-coloured liquid wax, with a faint, slightly sweet smell. This wax is obtained by crushing the jojoba seeds.

THERAPEUTIC PROPERTIES

Jojoba is beneficial for all skin types. It can be used alone, or blended 50:50 with sweet almond oil. It nourishes dry skin and is good for mature or elderly skin. It also contains an anti-inflammatory agent. As such it can be used on its own for gentle massage of arthritic or rheumatic joints, or for skin inflamed with dermatitis. It is helpful for dry scalps, and also for chapped skin, diaper rash or sunburn.

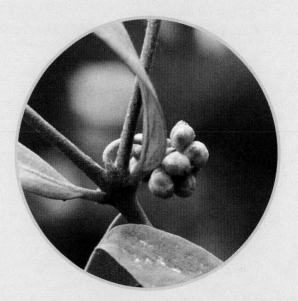

Calendula oil *(Calendula officinalis)*

Calendula oil comes from the marigold plant, which originated in the Mediterranean and has been cultivated since the Middle Ages for its pretty orange flowers. It now grows all over the world. The oil is obtained by maceration, meaning that the flowers are steeped in a vegetable oil, often organic sunflower oil, that has been stabilized against rancidity. The therapeutic constituents within the flowers are released into the vegetable oil, which is then used for massage. Like all macerated oils, the resulting product is expensive, but you can use calendula oil mixed 50:50 with sweet almond. This not only reduces cost but combines the effects of both oils. Calendula oil is pale yellow-orange in colour, with little aroma.

THERAPEUTIC PROPERTIES

Calendula is a gentle, healing oil, and is helpful in a blend for eczema, dermatitis or any dry, itchy skin condition. It can be beneficial when used alone on small areas, such as facial broken veins, or on a baby's bottom to heal diaper rash.

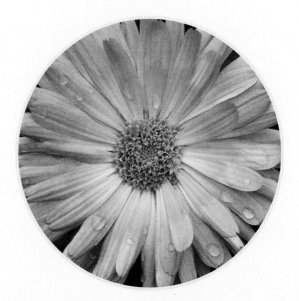

Avocado oil *(Persea gratissima)*

The avocado tree originates from the tropical and sub-tropical areas of the Americas. It is now cultivated in many countries, particularly Spain and Israel. Avocado oil is expressed from dried avocado pears that have been damaged and so cannot be sold as fresh fruit. The cosmetics industry uses a great deal of refined avocado oil; but for massage the unrefined, green, cold-pressed oil is preferred for its valuable therapeutic properties. It may appear slightly cloudy, with a faint avocado aroma.

THERAPEUTIC PROPERTIES

Avocado oil is a superb emollient, and is said to have a higher degree of penetration into the epidermis than most vegetable oils. As such, it is a particularly good carrier of essential oils. It is moisturising and softening, and especially recommended for dry or mature skin, or skin inclined to inflammation. As the unrefined, cold-pressed oil is expensive, it can be mixed 50:50 with sweet almond oil when you need a particularly rich oil.

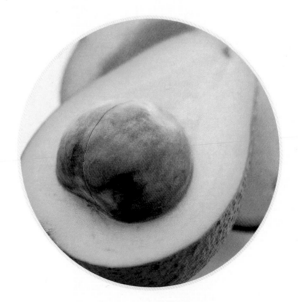

Evening primrose oil (*Oenothera biennis*)

Evening primrose is an edible plant, native to North America, that has long been used for its medicinal properties. It was introduced to Europe in 1619, and is now common throughout the Mediterranean. Its bright yellow flowers burst into bloom in early evening and then quickly die. They then form pods containing tiny seeds; these seeds are expressed, giving a pale yellow oil with little aroma.

THERAPEUTIC PROPERTIES

This oil is helpful for dry, scaly skin and for people with psoriasis or eczema. It is reputed to accelerate wound healing, but as new scar tissue must not be massaged, it should be used for massage only elsewhere on the body.

Blend it 50:50 with a nourishing oil such as jojoba for facial massage of mature skin. This combines the benefits of both oils.

Note: Evening primrose oil is highly unsaturated and so it is less stable than most other oils: it oxidizes if it is exposed to air or light. Buy it in small quantities and keep in a cool, dark place.

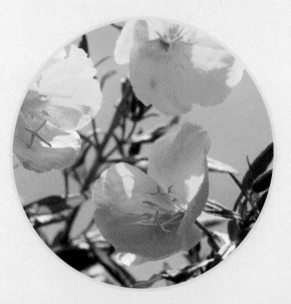

Peach kernel oil (*Prunus persica*)

The peach is a small tree up to 5m (15ft) tall, originating from China. Alexander the Great found it in Persia in the 4th century BCE, and by the 1st century CE, the Romans, who brought peaches to Europe, were calling the fruit "Persian apples". Although the peach was not introduced to America until the 17th century, California and Texas are now the world's major producers. The best-quality oil is obtained by cold-pressing the peach kernels, and produces a pale oil with no aroma.

THERAPEUTIC PROPERTIES

Peach kernel oil is particularly helpful for sensitive, dry or ageing skin, and can be used on its own for facial massage. As it is non-sensitizing, it makes an excellent choice for anyone who is prone to bad skin reactions. It is particularly emollient and nourishing to the skin. Peach kernel oil also relieves itching; so it is one of several useful oils that can be used on someone who suffers from eczema or dermatitis, where the skin is dry and irritated.

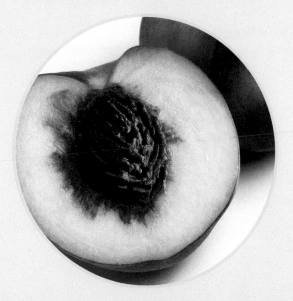

Rosehip oil (*Rosa canina*)

Rosa canina is known as the dog rose. The plant grows wild in the Andes, principally in Chile and Peru. It has white and pink flowers that ultimately form hips. Around 70% of the weight of the rose hips is made up of seeds; it is the seeds that are the source of the oil. These are cold-pressed to produce a golden-reddish oil, with a faint castor-oil aroma.

THERAPEUTIC PROPERTIES

Rosehip oil is helpful for skin regeneration, and has been found to prevent premature skin ageing. Blended 50:50 with jojoba oil it is wonderful for a facial massage for mature skin. Rosehip oil can also aid the formation of healthy scar tissue. Although you should not massage recent scar tissue, you can give rosehip oil to the person who is recovering to spread gently around the area to aid healing. It can also help skin inclined to eczema.

Note: Be sure to buy rosehip oil that is meant for massage – crude rosehip oil is produced by solvent extraction, and is not suitable.

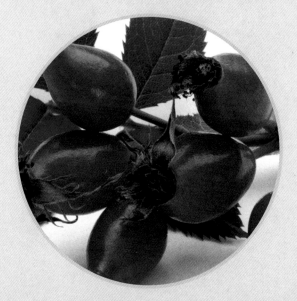

Wheat germ oil *(Triticum vulgare)*

Wheat is a cereal grass originating in western Asia but now widely cultivated in subtropical and temperate regions of the world. The stems, up to 1m (3ft) high, each bear a head of up to a hundred flower clusters in vertical rows. The oil is extracted from the wheat germ that makes up just 3% of each grain. The germ is stirred with a cold-pressed vegetable oil, which it soaks up. This product is then cold-pressed again, and yields a macerated oil made up of around one third wheat germ oil and two thirds vegetable oil. It is golden with a strong "wheaty" smell.

THERAPEUTIC PROPERTIES

Wheat germ oil is rich in lipid soluble vitamins, which makes it helpful for revitalizing dry skin.

It is also thought to help dermatitis; and it is beneficial for tired muscles, so could be included in a blend for use after exercise. Wheat germ is quite a viscous oil, so try blending it 50:50 with sweet almond oil.

Note: Anyone allergic to wheat flour should avoid this oil, as it could cause a skin reaction.

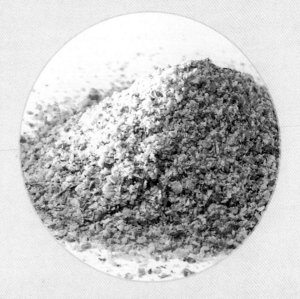

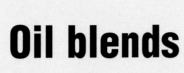

Oil blends

For information regarding essential oil safety and for guidelines on making your own massage blends, see pages 126 to 129.

CALMING AND RELAXING BLEND (2% dilution)
This is a particularly good stress-reliever and can also help battle insomnia.

Essential oils:
3 drops Roman chamomile (*Anthemis nobilis*)
3 drops Sweet marjoram (*Origanum majorana*)
2 drops Lavender (*Lavandula officinalis*)

Carrier oil:
4tsp (20ml) sweet almond

DECONGESTANT BLEND (2% dilution)
For the symptomatic relief of head colds and blocked sinuses.

Essential oils:
2 drops Eucalyptus (*Eucalyptus globulus*)
1 drop Tea tree (*Melaleuca alternifolia*)
1 drop Frankincense (*Boswellia carterii*)

Carrier oil:
2tsp (10ml) sweet almond

RELAXING AND COOLING BLEND (2% dilution)
This blend can be used to help with headaches, or in a foot massage to relieve any aching or tired feet.

Essential oils:
2 drops Lavender (*Lavandula officinalis*)
2 drops Peppermint (*Mentha piperta*)

Carrier oil:
2tsp (10ml) sweet almond

STIMULATING AND DETOXIFYING BLEND (2% dilution)
A good blend to use if your massage partner has just been exercising.

Essential oils:
3 drop Sweet marjoram (*Origanum majorana*)
3 drops Rosemary (*Rosmarinus officinalis*)
2 drops Juniper berry (*Juniperis communis*)

Carrier oils:
1tsp (5ml) avocado
3tsp (15ml) sweet almond

SENSITIVE SKIN BLEND (1% dilution)
A good all-round blend for anyone suffering from sensitive skin conditions.

Essential oils:
2 drops Sandalwood (*Santalum album*)
1 drop Frankincense (*Boswellia carterii*)
1 drop Geranium (*Pelargonium graveolens*)

Carrier oils:
2tsp (10ml) peach kernel *or* calendula
2tsp (10ml) sweet almond

CALMING AND WARMING BLEND (2% dilution)
This blend can help someone to unwind, and can relieve symptoms of period pain.

Essential oils:
4 drops Sweet marjoram (*Origanum majorana*)
4 drops Roman chamomile (*Anthemis nobilis*)
2 drops either Jasmine (*Jasminum officinale*),
  Rose (*Rosa centifolia* or *Rosa damascena*) or
  Lavender (*Lavandula officinalis*)

Carrier oils:
2tsp (10ml) avocado
2tsp (10ml) sweet almond

CALMING AND ANTI-SPASMODIC BLEND (2% dilution)
This blend can help to ease the symptoms of nervous exhaustion or a nervous stomach.

Essential oils:
3 drops Clary sage (*Salvia sclarea*)
3 drops Roman chamomile (*Anthemis nobilis*)
2 drops either Neroli (*Citrus aurantium*) or
  Petitgrain (*Citrus aurantium*)*

Carrier oils:
2tsp (10ml) avocado
2tsp (10ml) sweet almond

INVIGORATING AND STIMULATING BLEND (2% dilution)
A good blend to use if you are massaging someone before they do exercise, or if they are suffering from constipation.

Essential oils:
4 drops Rosemary (*Rosmarinus officinalis*)
2 drops Black pepper (*Piper nigrum*)
2 drops Bitter orange (*Citrus aurantium*)*

Carrier oils:
4tsp (20ml) sweet almond

*Bitter orange, neroli and petitgrain all share the same botanical name, but they come from different parts of the plant.

Bibliography

Harding, Jennie *Aromatherapy Massage for You*,
Duncan Baird Publishers (London), 2005

Harrold, Fiona *The Massage Manual*, Headline Book
Publishing (London) 1992

Leboyer, Frederick *Loving Hands: The Traditional Art
of Baby Massage*, Newmarket Press (New York), 1997

Maxwell-Hudson, Clare *Aromatherapy Massage Book*,
Dorling Kindersley (London), 1994

Price, Len *Carrier Oils for Aromatherapy and
Massage*, Riverhead (Stratford-upon-Avon), 1999

Price, Shirley *Aromatherapy for Common Ailments*,
Gaia Books Ltd (London), 1991

Smith, Karen *Massage: The Healing Power of Touch*,
Duncan Baird Publishers (London) 1999

Index

Acknowledgments

My thanks to everyone at DBP for producing books
so carefully and beautifully, especially to Becky Miles,
my editor; also to Matthew Ward the photographer and
Rachel Cross the designer. Thank you to Tamsin Mori as
well, for her helpful ideas.